# The Economics
# of Effective AIDS
# Treatment

Health, Nutrition, and Population Series

# The Economics of Effective AIDS Treatment

*Evaluating Policy Options for Thailand*

Ana Revenga,
Mead Over,
Emiko Masaki,
Wiwat Peerapatanapokin,
Julian Gold,
Viroj Tangcharoensathien,
Sombat Thanprasertsuk

With a Foreword by Sombat Thanprasertsuk,
M.D., Ministry of Public Health, Thailand

With contributions from Tim Brown, Chris Duncombe,
Jongkol Lertiendumrong, Seri Phongphit,
Bussaba Tantisak, and David Wilson

**THE WORLD BANK**
Washington, DC

ISBN-10: 0-8213-6755-2          eISBN: 0-8213-6756-0
ISBN-13: 978-0-8213-6755-1      DOI: 10.1596/978-0-8213-6755-1

*Library of Congress Cataloging-in-Publication Data has been applied for.*

# Contents

# Boxes, Figures, Maps, and Tables

## Boxes

## Figures

## Maps

## Tables

# Dedication

This report is dedicated to Nicholas Prescott, former staff member of the World Bank, who collaborated with the Thai government and the World Health Organization from 1995 through 1997 in an early analysis of the costs and benefits of antiretroviral therapy. Nicholas Prescott was a friend and mentor to many of the members of the current report team before his untimely death on February 19, 2000.

# Foreword

We in the National AIDS Prevention and Problem Alleviation Program of the Kingdom of Thailand bear the responsibility for managing national and non-national resources that are spent on protecting people from being infected with HIV and to provide care and treatment for the people who have already been infected. In this capacity, we are constantly aware of the need to balance the resources used for one aspect against those for another. Like officials in public health programs in other countries, we often have difficulty justifying expenditures to prevent disease when there are such clear and urgent needs all around us for treatment of people who are already sick. This is because well people are seldom aware that they have been saved from illness or death by a prevention expenditure made years previously by the Program. On the other hand, people who have been treated and are recovering attribute their recovery to those who helped them. It is more obvious and popular for a government to provide treatment than to provide prevention.

Although the subject matter of this book is the economics of AIDS treatment, perhaps its most important lessons are in the area of prevention. After carefully computing the probable future cost of Thailand's ARV treatment program, the authors have been able to compare that cost to the much larger cost that Thailand would have had to shoulder if the country had not engaged in such a vigorous HIV prevention program in the 1990s. They estimate that for every Baht that the Thai government spent on HIV prevention in the 1990s, 43 Baht of government expenditure on treatment has been avoided. Even if they have underestimated by 50 percent the cost of prevention (for example, by leaving out the value of the many voluntary contributions to HIV prevention of the members of many national NGOs) and overestimated the savings by a factor of two (because some of the reduction in risk behavior might have occurred without government intervention), one would estimate a saving of 10 Baht for every Baht spent on prevention. These calculations demonstrate the value of prevention of HIV and suggest that prevention of other diseases that afflict the nation might also be worthwhile investments.

This study forecasts that government spending on ARV therapy through the National Access to ARV for People with HIV and AIDS (NAPHA) will rise to equal 24 percent of the projected government health budget in the year 2013. But costs will rise even more if the availability of treatment leads to a return of high-risk behavior. The threat of these future costs has led to decisions by the National AIDS Committee early in 2006 to refocus on HIV prevention. In a speech at the United Nations General Assembly in New York in June 2006, Thailand announced that its new goal is to reduce by half the previously expected annual number of new HIV infections by the year 2010. To meet this goal, all stakeholders, including the government agencies and its civil society partners, will work together to sustain condom use where it is high and to increase it where it is low. New free condom distribution programs will be targeted to those particularly likely to contract and transmit HIV, including the discordant couples, female sex workers and their clients, intravenous drug users, men who have sex with men, clients of VCT and STI clinics, and youth as a cross-sectional group.

In view of the large cost of second-line drugs at current prices, the ARV Program is working with partners such as the Global Fund and Médecins sans Frontières to maximize the benefits of first-line therapy for each patient. As recommended in this study, we are expanding the coverage of patient support groups attached to each public antiretroviral treatment center.

We in the National AIDS Prevention and Problem Alleviation Program appreciate that the estimates in this book, although based on the best current information about costs and effects, are subject to change over time. The analytical framework used will be useful as we periodically return to these issues and construct new forecasts based on the most recent information. We look forward to future collaboration with the World Bank in the analysis of selected health sector policy issues.

*Sombat Thanprasertsuk, M.D., M.P.H.*
*Director, Bureau of AIDS, Tuberculosis,*
*and Sexually Transmitted Infections*

# Acknowledgments

This report was prepared by a joint study team from the World Bank and the Thailand Ministry of Public Health (MOPH). The team includes Sombat Thanprasertsuk and Cheewanan Lertpiriyasuwat (MOPH); Ana Revenga, Mead Over, and Emiko Masaki (World Bank); Tim Brown and Wiwat Peerapatanapokin (East-West Center); Viroj Tangcharoensathien and Jongkol Lertiendumrong (International Health Policy Program); Julian Gold and Chris Duncombe (HIV-NAT, Thai Red Cross), David Wilson and Nathan Ford (Médecins sans Frontières); and Seri Phongphit (Village Foundation). Excellent support and research assistance to the study team was provided by Nantaporn Ieumwananonthachai, Tasanee Chokwatana, Esther Rodriguez, Bussaba Tantisak, Chawewan Yenjtr, Sripen Tantivej, and Yumiko Kura.

The team would like to thank Siripen Supakakunti and her coauthors for sharing their early results on costing of antiretroviral therapy with the study team. The team also thanks Martha Ainsworth, Peter Heywood, Joan MacNeil, Elizabeth King, Patrick Brenny, Paul Toh, and participants in workshops in Washington, DC, and Bangkok for their useful comments and feedback.

The report was prepared under the guidance of Fadia Saadah (sector manager for health, nutrition, and population); Emmanuel Jimenez (sector director for human development); and Ian Porter (country director for Thailand). The team is especially grateful to Debrework Zewdie, director of the World Bank's Global AIDS Program, for her support throughout the preparation of this report.

# Abbreviations

| | |
|---|---|
| 3TC | Lamivudine |
| AEM | Asian Epidemiological Model |
| AIDS | Acquired immunodeficiency syndrome |
| ART | Antiretroviral therapy |
| ARV | Antiretroviral |
| ATC | Access to care |
| AZT | Zidovudine |
| BSS | Behavioral Surveillance Survey |
| CD4 | Immune cell that is a target for HIV (also called *T-cell*) |
| CMV | Cytomegalovirus |
| CRN | Clinical research network |
| CSMBS | Civil Servant Medical Benefit Scheme |
| d4T | Stavudine |
| ddI | Didanosine |
| DOTS | Directly observed treatment short course |
| EFV | Efavirenz |
| GFATM | Global Fund to Fight AIDS, Tuberculosis, and Malaria |
| GPO | Government Pharmaceutical Organization |
| HAART | Highly active antiretroviral therapy |
| HIV | Human immunodeficiency virus |
| HIV-NAT | HIV–Netherlands Australia Thailand Research Collaboration |
| IDU | Injecting drug user |
| IDV | Indinavir |
| IRS | Immune reconstitution syndrome |
| LPV | Lopinavir |
| LPV/r | Lopinavir/ritonavir |

| MAC | Mycobacterium avium complex |
|---|---|
| MDR-TB | Multidrug-resistant TB |
| MOPH | Ministry of Public Health |
| MSF | Médecins sans Frontières |
| MSM | Men who have sex with men |
| NAPHA | National Access to Antiretroviral Program for People Living with HIV/AIDS |
| NESDB | National Economic and Social Development Board |
| NGO | Nongovernmental organization |
| NNRTI | Nonnucleoside reverse transcriptase inhibitor |
| NRTI | Nucleoside reverse transcriptase inhibitor |
| NVP | Nevirapine |
| OECD | Organisation for Economic Co-operation and Development |
| OI | Opportunistic infection |
| PCP | Pneumocystis carinii pneumonia |
| PHA | Person living with HIV/AIDS |
| PI | Protease inhibitor |
| PMTCT | Prevention of mother-to-child transmission |
| RTV | Ritonavir |
| SGOT | Serum glutamic oxaloacetic transaminase |
| SQV | Saquinavir |
| SQV/r | Saquinavir/ritonavir |
| SSS | Social Security Scheme |
| STI | Sexually transmitted infection |
| TB | Tuberculosis |
| TNP+ | Thai Network of People Living with AIDS |
| TRIPS | Agreement on Trade-Related Aspects of Intellectual Property Rights |
| UCS | Universal Coverage Scheme |
| UNAIDS | Joint United Nations Programme on HIV/AIDS |
| VCT | Voluntary counseling and testing |
| WCF | Workmen's Compensation Fund |
| WHO | World Health Organization |
| WTO | World Trade Organization |

# Executive Summary

## Background

Thailand is in the vanguard of developing countries that are seeking to provide antiretroviral therapy (ART) as the standard of care to large numbers of people with symptomatic HIV disease. As of May 2006, 77,758 people living with HIV/AIDS in Thailand had received ART through the National Access to Antiretroviral Program for People Living with HIV/AIDS (or NAPHA), and approximately 8,000 are estimated to have access to ART through the Social Security Scheme. The Thai government's objective is to provide ART to 82,000 people living with HIV/AIDS by end of fiscal year 2006.

The purpose of this report is to advise the Thai government and Thai society at large about the full range of benefits, costs, and consequences that are likely to result from the decision to expand public provision of ART through NAPHA and to assist with the design of implementation policies that will achieve maximum treatment benefits, while promoting prevention of HIV/AIDS and maintaining financial sustainability within Thailand.

### Provision of ART in Thailand

The first case of AIDS in Thailand was reported in September 1984. Since then, more than 1 million Thais have been infected with HIV, and, of those, more than 400,000 have died. In 2004, an estimated 572,500 Thais were living with HIV/AIDS (table ES.1). Among those people, some 49,500 will develop serious AIDS-related illnesses during the year, and about the same number will die of AIDS-related complications. It is also estimated that 19,500 new infections will occur in 2004 (compared with 143,000 new infections in 1990 and 23,676 new infections in 2002).

The Royal Thai government and Thai society have demonstrated a strong commitment to providing comprehensive care and support to persons living with HIV/AIDS (PHAs), but it is only recently that they have been able to provide ART to large numbers of people with symptomatic HIV (figure ES.1). The availability of a domestically produced triple-drug combination, GPO-vir,[1] at affordable prices (about B 1,200, or US$30 per month) has opened the door for many PHAs, who could previously not afford ART, to have access to it, as well as allowing the Ministry of Public Health (MOPH) to roll out a large-scale

**Table ES.1** Estimated Cumulative Numbers of HIV/AIDS, 2004

|  | Cumulative number |
| --- | --- |
| Total HIV infections (adults and children) | 1,074,155 |
| Total deaths (adults and children) | 501,600 |
| People living with HIV | 572,484 |
| Projected new HIV infections in 2004 | 19,471 |
| Projected new AIDS cases in 2004 | 49,542 |

Source: Thai Working Group on HIV/AIDS Projections for 2004.

**Figure ES.1** Access to HIV/AIDS Medical Care in Thailand

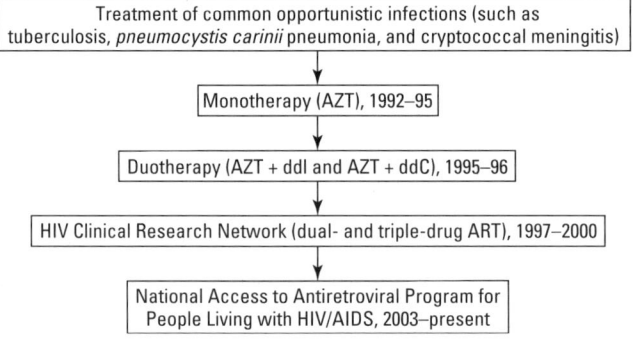

Source: MOPH 2004.

campaign to provide triple-drug ART as standard care. As a result, the number of PHAs on ART has increased sharply from about 3,000 at the start of 2002 to 27,000 by the end of 2003, rising to 52,593 by February 2005. The program is financed in part by the Global Fund to Fight AIDS, Tuberculosis, and Malaria (GFATM) and, in part, by the government budget. The number of treatment sites increased from 112 in 2001 to 462 in early 2003, rising to 841 by February 2005.

Table ES.2 shows the evolution of estimated cases of PHAs, estimates of AIDS cases, and numbers of people having access to public ART in Thailand. As of the end of 2004, more than 80 percent of those living with AIDS had access to public ART—a remarkable achievement.

### Benefits of Prior Prevention Efforts

Successful implementation of NAPHA poses a significant challenge to the Royal Thai government and to Thai society. In a few years, as AIDS patients live longer with ART, the health system will need to provide care not only to 10,000 to 20,000 new cases per year, but also to most of those whose lives have been significantly prolonged by ART. Given the commitment across all segments of Thai society, the country's significant health system capacity, and the availability of internal and external financing, Thailand has good prospects for meeting this challenge. Its ability to even contemplate providing care to all those who need it, however, rests on the success of its past prevention efforts.

In the absence of past successful efforts of national prevention, HIV infections—and, hence, AIDS cases—today would be much higher than they actually are (figure ES.2). We have estimated that without such efforts, Thailand would have 7.7 million HIV cases and 850,000 AIDS cases in 2005, roughly 14 times more of each than exist in reality. If we suppose that Thailand would try to offer ART to all of this much larger number of AIDS patients, its budget requirements would also be 14 times greater and would continue to grow over the next decade. Thanks to its substantial prevention efforts between 1991 and 2002, Thailand has avoided the need to spend an additional US$18.6 billion (B 745 billion) on treatment over the decade through 2012.

During the 1990s, Thailand spent more than most countries on its HIV/AIDS program. Its total budget expenditure on prevention and treatment combined over this period was a substantial US$434 million

**Table ES.2**  Estimated Cases of People Living with HIV/AIDS, AIDS Cases, Reported AIDS Cases in Public Hospitals, and Access to Public ART

| | 1997 | 1998 | 1999 | 2000 | 2001 | 2002 | 2003 | 2004 |
|---|---|---|---|---|---|---|---|---|
| People living with HIV/AIDS (projected) | 751,235 | 740,349 | 719,765 | 649,564 | 665,344 | 635,057 | 603,942 | 572,484 |
| People living with AIDS (projected) | 59,752 | 65,333 | 68,311 | 68,677 | 67,057 | 64,832 | 62,871 | 61,394 |
| Patients in public ART (projected) | 1,095[a] | 1,095[a] | 1,095[a] | 2,095[a] | 2,095[a] | 8,341[a] | 27,158 | 52,593[b] |
| Actual persons in public ART as a percentage of projected AIDS cases | 1.8 | 1.7 | 1.6 | 3.1 | 3.1 | 12.9 | 43.2 | 81.4 |
| Actual persons in public ART as a percentage of actual reported AIDS cases | 4.1 | 4.0 | 4.0 | 4.5 | 8.5 | 35.5 | 122.6 | — |

*Sources:* The Thai Working Group on HIV/AIDS Projection 2001. Projections for HIV/AIDS in Thailand: 2000–2020, Karnsana printing press. Gold and others 2005. The data on Reported AIDS cases accessed to public care are provided by MOPH 2004; UNAIDS 2002.

*Note:* — = not available.

a. This figure comes from UNAIDS 2002.

b. This figure is for February 2005.

**Figure ES.2** Importance of Prior Prevention Efforts

*Source:* Brown and Peerapatanapokin 2004.

in 2002 dollars (B 17.3 billion). However, by averting the need to spend US$18.6 billion (B 745 billion) over the subsequent decade, each dollar (or baht) invested in the 1990s saved US$43 (or B 1720) in needed treatment expenditure in the subsequent decade. It is doubtful that any other Thai government investment achieved such a high benefit-cost ratio. The finance ministries of countries such as China and India, where the HIV/AIDS epidemic is at an earlier stage, should be aware of the high return to HIV/AIDS prevention campaigns when they make intersectoral allocations of their governments' budgets.

Even in Thailand, however, there is no room for complacency. Although policies have been successful in lowering new infections, prevalence of HIV in high-risk groups is still high—especially among those groups that past prevention efforts did not explicitly target, such as intravenous drug users (IDUs) or male sex workers. There is also evidence that the effect of past prevention campaigns is waning. Recent rounds of the Behavioral Surveillance Survey (BSS) show that the percentage of male conscripts reporting sexual relationships with commercial sex workers, after declining for several years, has started to increase again in 2002 and 2003. The same pattern is visible with other female sex partners and among married conscripts who have extramarital sex. Condom use among those male conscripts is not high: only 59 percent report consistent use of condoms with sex workers, and only 25 percent do so with nonregular female sex partners. New risk behaviors by other groups, such as youth, also need to be addressed.

## Measurement of the Effect of ART Policy

Because the objective of ART policy is to lengthen and improve the lives of the recipients, a natural measure of the effectiveness of a policy is the number of life-years that ART adds to the population. Public policy makers need to consider not only the direct effects of ART policy on the patients receiving ART, but also the indirect effects of ART on the creation of new HIV infections. For example, increasing evidence suggests that ART patients are significantly less infectious than they would be in the absence of ART or with only mono- or duotherapy. However, growing evidence also indicates that greater access to ART may lead to complacency and increased risk behavior by people on ART and by people (whether HIV negative or positive) in surrounding communities (Dukers and others 2001; Stolte and others 2001; Van de Ven 2005).

Assessing the spillover effects of ART on people other than the patient is an indispensable part of designing a policy. Table ES.3 provides a classification of the indirect (or external) effects into biological and behavioral effects on transmission. Within each of the categories, the effects could be beneficial by slowing transmission or could be

**Table ES.3**  Possible Effects of ART on HIV Transmission

| | | Direction of effect | |
| --- | --- | --- | --- |
| | | Beneficial (slow transmission) | Adverse (speedy transmission) |
| Type of effect | Biological | Reduces infectiousness. ART may lower viral loads and may therefore lower the risk of transmission per sexual contact. | Selects for resistance. Imperfect adherence to ART selects for resistant strains of the virus, which can then be transmitted. Longer duration of infectivity. The greater longevity of HIV infected people taking ART has the unintended negative consequence of increasing the period during which the patient can transmit the virus. |
| | Behavioral | Encourages prevention, especially diagnostic testing. ART may increase the uptake rates of prevention activities, particularly voluntary counseling and testing. | Increases risk behavior. People receiving ART, and HIV positives and negatives in the surrounding community, may engage in more risky behaviors than they would if ART were unavailable. |

Source: Over and others 2004.

adverse by accelerating it. The measure of the importance of any of those effects is the rate of new HIV infections, or the *HIV incidence rate.*

To project the costs of ART policy, we have adopted the simplifying assumption that most program costs will be related to the individual patient in the form of provider time, pharmaceutical products, diagnostic tests, and disposable paper and rubber products. Therefore, the costs will not vary much with scale or scope. The exception we are making to this rule is the cost of equipping a health care facility that is not a district hospital with the capacity to administer ART. We assume that to qualify to manage one or more ART patients, any facility must train a minimum number of providers in ART protocols, and that to keep providers abreast of the rapidly changing technology of ART, the facility must retrain those staff members every year. This category of costs might be called *recurrent fixed costs.* The costs recur every year as a function of the number of facilities but can be spread over all the patients at the facility.

### The Effects of Thailand's ART Policy

To estimate the effect of NAPHA and then of the cost-effectiveness of various modifications of NAPHA, we must model how the specific changes introduced by NAPHA influence the behavior of patients and providers. Our approach is to construct a model of the links between government instruments and policy outcomes. We do this in five steps summarized in figure ES.3.

- First, we model the link from the two primary policy instruments—price and availability (or supply)—to the distribution of patient demand for care.

- Second, we project the evolution of prices and availability into the future, and we then compute the projected distribution of demand across treatment options.

- Third, we apply the expected demand to the Thai population of eligible infected people, as projected by an updated version of the Asian Epidemiological Model (AEM),[2] in order to deduce the future of ART use.

**Figure ES.3** Policies to Epidemiology to Performance

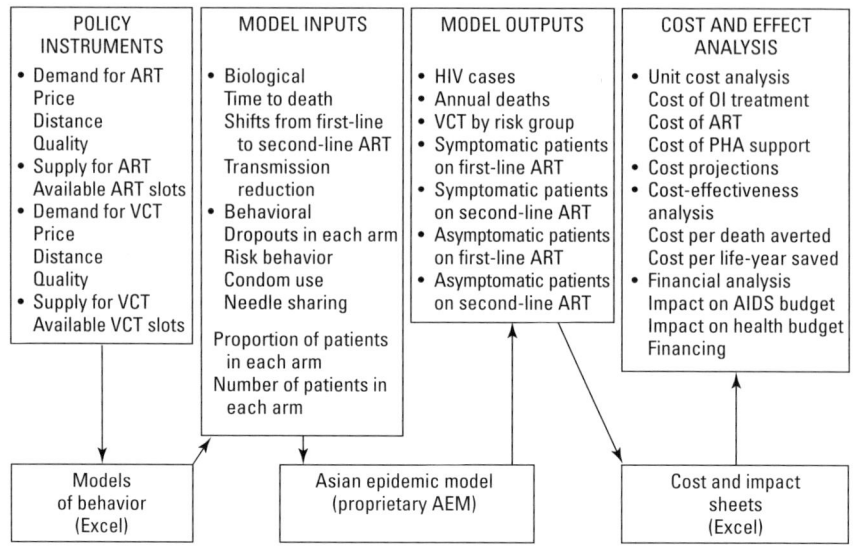

| POLICY INSTRUMENTS | MODEL INPUTS | MODEL OUTPUTS | COST AND EFFECT ANALYSIS |
|---|---|---|---|
| • Demand for ART<br>  Price<br>  Distance<br>  Quality<br>• Supply for ART<br>  Available ART slots<br>• Demand for VCT<br>  Price<br>  Distance<br>  Quality<br>• Supply for VCT<br>  Available VCT slots | • Biological<br>  Time to death<br>  Shifts from first-line<br>   to second-line ART<br>  Transmission<br>   reduction<br>• Behavioral<br>  Dropouts in each arm<br>  Risk behavior<br>  Condom use<br>  Needle sharing<br><br>Proportion of patients<br> in each arm<br>Number of patients in<br> each arm | • HIV cases<br>• Annual deaths<br>• VCT by risk group<br>• Symptomatic patients<br>  on first-line ART<br>• Symptomatic patients<br>  on second-line ART<br>• Asymptomatic patients<br>  on first-line ART<br>• Asymptomatic patients<br>  on second-line ART | • Unit cost analysis<br>  Cost of OI treatment<br>  Cost of ART<br>  Cost of PHA support<br>• Cost projections<br>• Cost-effectiveness<br>  analysis<br>  Cost per death averted<br>  Cost per life-year saved<br>• Financial analysis<br>  Impact on AIDS budget<br>  Impact on health budget<br>  Financing |

| Models of behavior (Excel) | Asian epidemic model (proprietary AEM) | Cost and impact sheets (Excel) |
|---|---|---|

*Source:* Authors.

• Fourth, we estimate the direct and spillover effects of ART use on health and HIV incidence.

• Fifth, we apply unit costs to estimate the financial burden of the NAPHA policy.

### *Projection Scenarios*

The effect of a policy choice can be defined only in comparison to what would have happened in the absence of this choice. This alternative scenario, called a *baseline* or *counterfactual,* is a projection of the future course of AIDS treatment if the Royal Thai government had not introduced its expanded NAPHA program. Several alternative baseline scenarios could have been chosen—see cells (a), (b) and (c) in table ES.4. Each of these scenarios corresponds to a different combination of public financing of ART and government subsidization of the production and sale of low-cost ART. The chosen baseline corresponds to cell (a): what would have happened if the government had kept only its previously existing (pre-2001) voluntary program, with only branded drugs available?

**Table ES.4** Potential Baseline Scenarios or Counterfactuals to NAPHA

| | | Government to finance ART publicly | |
|---|---|---|---|
| | | No (private out-of-pocket only) | Yes |
| Government to produce and sell low-cost ART (GPO-vir) | No | (A) Baseline scenario: No government intervention takes place. There is a voluntary program only, too small to make a difference. | (B) Government provides subsidized public production with no possibility of alternative supply channels (buyers' clubs and so forth). |
| | Yes | (C) GPO produces and markets GPO-vir at current prices (less than US$1 per day), but government does not expand public delivery of ART through the public health system beyond the voluntary Access to Care program. | (D) NAPHA: This scenario includes the current form and alternative versions including stimulating VCT for earlier recruitment and introducing demand-side incentives to increase adherence. |

*Source:* Authors.

The effect of NAPHA is obtained by comparing outcomes from cell (A) to those from cell (D). The total effect could be separated into one part because of the availability of low-cost generic ART and another part as a result of the public finance of ART provision. Such a deconstruction would enable us to attribute some portions of the benefits of NAPHA to each of its two components and another portion to the synergy between them. We do not undertake that deconstruction here.

In addition to the NAPHA policy scenario described above, the report considers two enhancements to NAPHA and a third policy that

**Table ES.5** Policy Scenarios for the NAPHA Program

| | | Encourage VCT and Early Recruitment into ART | |
|---|---|---|---|
| | | No | Yes |
| Encourage adherence through demand-side incentives such as PHA groups, accompagnateurs, and conditional transfers | No | NAPHA (D1): Current implementation of NAPHA program (recruitment of mainly symptomatic HIV through the public health system) | VCT (D2): Earlier recruitment through VCT (at higher CD4 counts), without improved adherence |
| | Yes | Adherence (D3): Improved adherence without earlier recruitment (keep current recruitment of symptomatic HIV through public health system) | VCT and Adherence (D4): Improved adherence and earlier recruitment (recruit earlier through VCT at higher CD4 counts) |

*Source:* Authors.

would combine those two enhancements (table ES.5). The enhancements are chosen to address what are perceived by knowledgeable Thai and international observers to be potential weak points in the NAPHA program and, indeed, in all publicly financed and publicly provided ART programs worldwide.

Early analyses of the general effectiveness and cost-effectiveness of publicly provided ART assumed that many HIV-infected patients would be recruited to treatment when their immune systems first dropped below an eligibility threshold. As a result, the benefits of ART would be maximized. However, experience in Thailand, as well as in several other countries (for example, Botswana, Brazil, Malawi, and member states of the Organisation for Economic Co-operation and Development), shows that most patients are identified as being ART eligible only when their opportunistic illnesses lead them to the hospital, which is usually when their CD4 counts are already well below the threshold at which they would most benefit from care. Thus, it is useful to analyze an alternative version of NAPHA that would include a much more vigorous promotion of voluntary counseling and testing (VCT) in an effort to attract patients into treatment when they first become eligible for it.

A major challenge for ART programs will be to attain and sustain high levels of adherence among their patients. Ministry-sponsored training programs for public sector ART providers are currently teaching the importance of adherence. However, experience around the world suggests that, as ART treatment is scaled up, it will be increasingly difficult to attain high levels of adherence among new patients and to sustain those levels among all patients. One promising approach with which Thailand has already experimented is both to subsidize and to facilitate the establishment of nongovernmental organizations that provide emotional, physical, and sometimes even financial support to patients. In this report, we refer to public sector delivery that has been strengthened by adding those demand-enhancing programs as augmented public delivery of ART. Our "Augmented (D3)" scenario is intended to capture the incremental benefits and costs of such a program.

We also model a "Both (D4)" program, which includes the costs both of expanded VCT and of augmented adherence and models a synergistic benefit between them.

## Costs of ART

Costs of ART can be defined in many ways, such as costs to the public sector, to individual patients, and to society. To evaluate the various policy options for expanding public provision of ART in Thailand, we adopt the perspective of and estimate the costs to the public sector. Average costs of ART per patient are estimated according to the types of treatment regimens (first-line therapy and second-line therapy); modes of service delivery (public, augmented public, and private service delivery); and stages of the disease (asymptomatic and symptomatic HIV). Specific cost components included in estimating average costs of ART per patient are costs of ARV drugs, lab tests, and monitoring; costs of treating opportunistic infections (OIs); and PHA support expenses. Cost data were obtained from existing studies in Thailand, both published and unpublished, and from informal consultations with local and international experts.

**Table ES.6**  Costs of ARV Drugs per Patient by Types of Regimens in Thailand

| | Monthly cost | | Annual cost | |
|---|---|---|---|---|
| *Antiretroviral drugs* | *Baht* | *US$* | *Baht* | *US$* |
| *First-line regimens (per MOPH guideline)* | | | | |
| (1) 3TC + d4T + nevirapine | 1,200 | 30.0 | 14,400 | 360.0 |
| (2) d4T + 3TC + efavirenz | 2,579 | 64.5 | 30,948 | 773.7 |
| AZT + 3TC + efavirenz | 3,819 | 95.5 | 45,828 | 1,145.7 |
| AZT + 3TC + nevirapine[a] | 2,400 | 60.0 | 28,800 | 720.0 |
| (3) d4T + 3TC + IDV/r | 3,500 | 87.5 | 42,000 | 1,050.0 |
| AZT + 3TC + IDV/r | 4,740 | 118.5 | 56,880 | 1,422.0 |
| Average cost | 1,606 | 40.1 | 19,271 | 481.80 |
| *Second-line regimens (per WHO guideline)* | | | | |
| ABC + ddI + LPV/r | 22,822 | 570.6 | 273,864 | 6,846.6 |
| ABC + ddI + SQV/r | 22,094 | 552.4 | 265,128 | 6,628.2 |
| Average cost | 22,458 | 561.5 | 269,496 | 6,737.4 |

*Sources:* Bureau of AIDS, Tuberculosis, and Sexually Transmitted Infections, MOPH, 2004; Duncombe 2004; GPO 2004.
*Note:* US$1 = B 40. Costs of ARV drugs are based on the lowest prices available (either generic or branded drugs) in Thailand, as of September 2004.
a. The GPO is currently in the process of producing a fixed-dose combination of GPO-Z (AZT, 3TC, and nevirapine). The cost of GPO-Z is approximately B 1,400 baht (US$35) per month.

**Table ES.7**  Annual Cost per Patient by Types of Drug Regimens

| Cost Items | | Annual cost per patient | | | |
| --- | --- | --- | --- | --- | --- |
| | | 1st line | | 2nd line | |
| | | Baht | US$ | Baht | US$ |
| (1) ARV drugs | | 18,847 | 471.2 | 263,567 | 6,589.2 |
| (2) Lab tests | | 1,210 | 30.3 | 1,210 | 30.3 |
| (3) OI treatment | | 4,815 | 120.4 | 4,815 | 120.4 |
| (4) OPD service | | 2,773 | 69.3 | 2,773 | 69.3 |
| (5) IPD service | | 6,041 | 151.0 | 6,041 | 151.0 |
| (6) ARVs + lab tests | (1) + (2) | 20,057 | 501.4 | 264,778 | 6,619.4 |
| (7) Hospital services (IPD+OPD) | (4) + (5) | 8,815 | 220.4 | 8,815 | 220.4 |
| (8) Total ART cost | (3)+(6)+(7) | 33,688 | 842.2 | 278,408 | 6,960.2 |

Source: Supakankunti and others 2004.
Note: The presented cost per patient is an average cost of provincial and community hospitals.
OPD- outpatient department
IPD – inpatient department

Table ES.6 summarizes costs of various regimens currently available and recommended by the Thai Ministry of Public Health (MOPH) and World Health Organization (WHO) in their treatment guidelines. The annual costs of ARV drugs vary significantly between first-line and second-line regimens, ranging from B 14,400 (using GPO-vir) to B 273,864 (using expensive protease inhibitors, or PIs) per patient per year. The average cost of first-line ART regimens is estimated at B 19,271 (US$481.80) per patient per year, using a weighted average of three categories of ART drug regimens under the MOPH treatment guideline.[3] The average cost of second-line regimens is estimated at B 270,000 (US$6,740) per patient, costing 14 times more than the average cost of first-line regimens.

In addition to the cost of ARV drugs, significant costs are associated with providing and monitoring ART treatment. The costs of outpatient and inpatient services are not negligible because uses of medical services increase at the time of initiating ART treatment. On the basis of the estimates above, the annual average cost of ART using first-line therapy is estimated at B 33,700 (US$840) per patient (table ES.7). The costs of ARV drugs and lab monitoring represent nearly 60 percent of the total ART expenses when first-line therapy is used, and the costs increase to 95 percent of the ART expenses when patients are on second-line therapy.

**Figure ES.4**   Cost-Effectiveness of NAPHA with First-Line ART Compared with NAPHA with Both First- and Second-Line ART

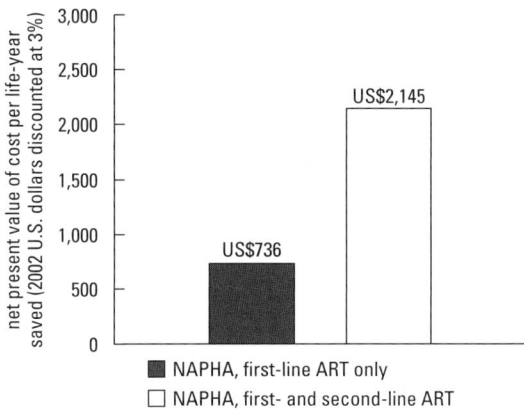

Source: Authors' construction.

## Main Findings

The study has several significant findings.

### Finding 1: NAPHA with First-Line Regimen Only Is the Most Cost-Effective Policy Option of Those Studied

NAPHA with first-line therapy only—at a cost of US$736 or B 29,440 per discounted life-year saved—is the most affordable and cost-effective policy option modeled in this report. Figure ES.4 presents the cost per life-year saved of NAPHA without second-line drugs when compared to the cost per life-year saved of NAPHA with second-line therapy. The central finding is that the NAPHA program with second-line drugs can save years of life for US$2,145, (B 85,800), whereas NAPHA with only first-line therapy is far more cost-effective at US$736 (B 29,440) per discounted life-year saved.

In the absence of significant change in the price of second-line drugs, the cost of saving an additional life-year through second-line therapy is high when compared to the substantial health benefits of first-line policy only. On a pure cost-effectiveness basis, a policy with first-line therapy only would be superior. However, other considerations may weigh heavily on the government's final decision as to what policy to adopt. From the perspective of this study, affordability and equity are also relevant criteria.

An argument for horizontal equity would compare NAPHA with and without second-line therapy to the cost of saving life-years through subsidized treatment of other adult illnesses, such as cancer, heart disease, or end-stage renal disease. This comparison would show that NAPHA with second-line therapy is cost-effective relative to those other interventions. Advocates of vertical equity would argue that the government should ensure that the bottom of the income distribution has access to care that the top one-fifth will purchase for themselves (including second-line therapy).

### Finding 2: NAPHA with Second-Line Therapy Is Still Affordable and Yields Large Benefits in Terms of Life-Years Saved

By 2015, the current NAPHA policy will have added about 220,000 people per year to the living population. Even at the end of the projection horizon, when the Thai AIDS epidemic is predicted to slow, the NAPHA policy will be saving about 190,000 life-years each year (figure ES.5). Hence,10 percent more life-years would be saved under the current NAPHA policy than under an equivalent NAPHA without second-line therapy. By keeping people alive longer, NAPHA will be associated with an increase in the number of HIV-infected people

**Figure ES.5**  Benefits (Life-Years Saved) and Costs of NAPHA relative to Baseline

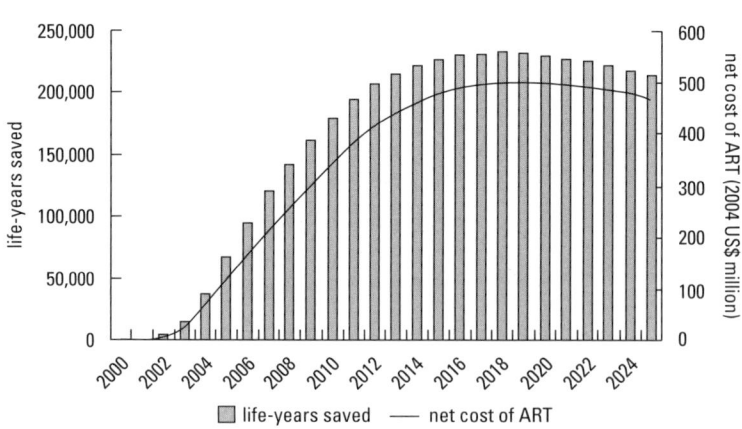

*Source:* Authors.

**Figure ES.6**  After 2010, Most Costs Are for Second-Line Therapy

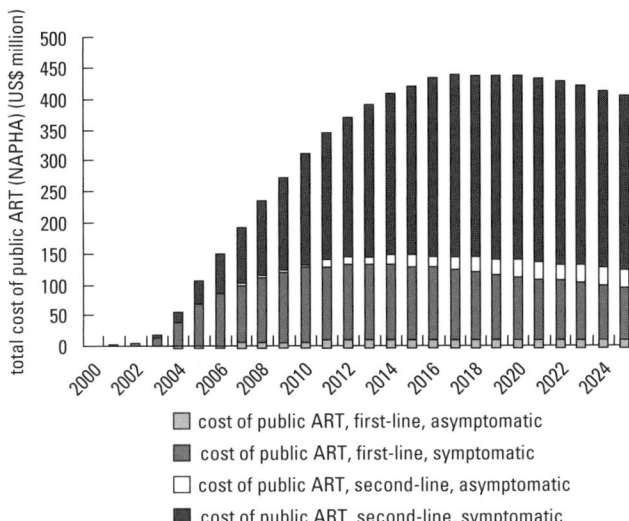

Source: Authors.
Note: The notation *symptomatic* refers to symptomatic patients whose CD4 counts are below 50 cells per cubic millimeter. The notation *asymptomatic* refers to asymptomatic patients whose CD4 counts are between 50 and 200 cells per cubic millimeter.

in Thailand, as well as with a significant increase in the number of people living with HIV/AIDS who are on treatment. As a result, prevalence rates will no longer be an adequate objective for national HIV strategy (because success in treatment will be tied to an increase in the prevalence rate).

The total cost of NAPHA with second-line therapy reaches a ceiling at US$500 million or B 20 billion per year in 2020. Beginning in 2008, expenditure on second-line therapy accounts for more than one-half of total ART spending. By the end of the projection, one-fourth of the patients receiving second-line therapy will absorb three-fourths of the treatment budget (figure ES.6). The projected cost of NAPHA will increase Thailand's AIDS spending from its current level of about US$100 million or B 4 billion per year to more than five times that amount in 2020. However, even at its peak, total spending on AIDS treatment will require increasing the total health care spending by less than 25 percent. We judge this level of expenditures to be affordable to the Thai government.

**Figure ES.7** Projected Annual Life-Years Saved under Alternative Scenarios Relative to Baseline

Source: Authors.

## *Finding 3: Policy Options to Enhance Adherence and to Recruit Patients Earlier Are a Good Public Investment*

Timely patient recruitment and enhanced adherence buy additional life-years. If initiated now, the expanded VCT, augmented adherence, and "both" policies would benefit more patients each year until the approaches save, respectively, 18,000, 50,000, and 60,000 additional life-years in 2020, on top of the 210,000 life-years saved that were generated by NAPHA alone in that year (figure ES.7). Thus, for 2020, the alternative policies offer the possibility of improving NAPHA benefits by almost 30 percent.

The expanded policies, however, also involve additional costs. Of the four policies considered, the current NAPHA policy is the most cost-effective (figure ES.8). The second-most cost-effective is the augmented treatment policy, which enhances patient adherence. We estimate that systematically adding patient support groups to all treatment sites in Thailand would increase the cost per life-year saved by less than US$40 (B 1,600), thereby making this approach a good investment. Under the central assumptions of the model, spending the resources on expanded HIV testing in order to recruit patients in a more timely manner would increase the cost per life-year saved by only another US$60 (B 2,400), which also seems like a good buy. Thus, we recommend that Thailand undertake both of the two analyzed policies to strengthen treatment, bringing the estimated cost per life-year saved to US$2,243 or B 89,720.[4]

**Figure ES.8**   Cost-Effectiveness of NAPHA and Alternative Scenarios Relative to Baseline

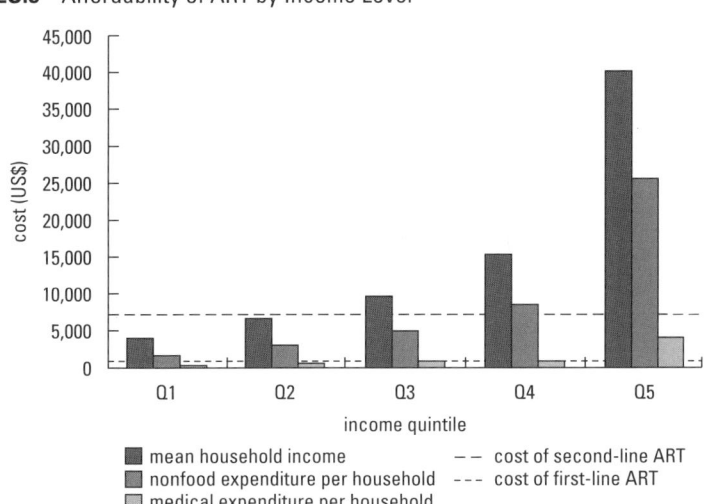

*Source:* Authors.

## Finding 4: Public Financing Will Help Ensure Equitable Access

Suppose that Thailand had reduced the price of first-line ART by authorizing the production of GPO-vir but had refrained from subsidizing treatment. For the top two quintiles in the income distribution, first-line ART could be affordable through user fees (figure ES.9). Even for the bottom two quintiles, the US$842 or B 33,680 cost of first-line therapy compares with the medical expenses of the sickest households for a single year. The problems for the poorest households are likely to be caused by two unusual features of the cost of treatment. First, the treatment must continue for the rest of the patient's

**Figure ES.9**   Affordability of ART by Income Level

*Source:* Authors.

life. For those households in the lowest 80 percent of the income distribution that are able to raise the resources to pay the US$842 for one year, the second and third year will become increasingly onerous. Second, poverty-induced laxity in treatment will lead to treatment failure, to development of resistant strains of the virus, to spread of those resistant strains to others, and to the requirement that the patient move to second-line therapy.

Although it is conceivable that the cost of first-line therapy could be partially financed with user fees, second-line therapy is much more expensive, exceeding the total household income of 40 percent of the population. Most people on first-line therapy will eventually need second-line therapy, and they will not be able to afford it without public support.

### Finding 5: Public Financing Can Strengthen Positive Spillovers and Can Limit Negative Spillovers of ART

ART may be used to increase the effectiveness of prevention activities, especially VCT. But this beneficial effect of ART requires greater integration of treatment and prevention efforts than currently exists in Thailand.

Poor adherence to first-line therapy will speed the development of viral resistance to those drugs and will hasten the day when the patient must move to second-line therapy. Public intervention to support adherence can limit the spread of resistant virus. From a social as well as an individual perspective, adherence support mechanisms such as the augmented public care that we model in this report are likely to be cost-effective as well as therapeutically beneficial.

### Finding 6: If the Success of ART Rollout Makes People or the Government Complacent about Prevention, Future Costs Could Rise Substantially

If the availability of ART is accompanied by a sustained government prevention program and if it leads people to reduce risk behaviors such as injecting drugs and having unprotected sex, then the cost-effectiveness of ART is improved by about 9 percent, and future government expenditures on ART will go down by US$926 million or B 37 billion, or by 14 percent.

**Figure ES.10**  Cost-Effectiveness of Main Scenarios compared with Disinhibition Scenario

*Source:* Authors.

Conversely, if the availability of ART crowds out government expenditure on prevention and leads people to increase their risk behavior back to its levels in the early 1980s, government treatment expenditure will increase more than threefold. In such a case, as shown in figure ES.10, the cost per life-year saved would increase nearly threefold, from US$2,145 to US$6,243 (from B 85,800 to B 249,720).

### Finding 7: Future Government Expenditures on ART and the Lives It Will Save Are Highly Sensitive to Negotiated Agreements on the Intellectual Property Rights for Pharmaceuticals

Because the drugs used in second-line therapy are patented, produced, and sold by multinational pharmaceutical corporations, Thailand must either pay the high prices demanded by those monopolies or exercise its rights under World Trade Organization (WTO) treaties to grant a compulsory license for the manufacture of the drug, subject to negotiated royalties.

Because Thailand stands to gain a great deal from bilateral agreements to reduce trade barriers with trading partners such as the United States, the Royal Thai government may be tempted to relinquish its rights to grant compulsory licenses for AIDS drugs in exchange for proffered trade advantages. The report finds that the cost of such concessions would be large. For example, by exercising compulsory licensing to reduce the cost of second-line therapy by 90 percent, the government would reduce its future budgetary obligations by US$3.2 billion discounted (B 127 billion discounted) through 2025 and would cut by more than half the cost per life-year saved of the NAPHA program, from US$2,145 to US$940 (or B 85,800 to B 37,600) per life-year saved.

The size of royalty payments that the WTO mandates to accompany compulsory licensing is indeterminate and is subject to negotiation. Thailand could enhance its bargaining power vis-à-vis the multinational pharmaceutical industry by coordinating its negotiations with other middle- and low-income countries.

## Conclusions and Recommendations

In its current form, Thailand's NAPHA program is affordable. Under the model's assumptions, it is also cost-effective relative to the baseline scenario. Furthermore, although the two enhanced policies we suggest (early recruitment through expanded VCT and improved adherence through PHA groups) are less cost-effective, they are still a good bargain, particularly if both are enacted.

Much of the cost of ART over the long term is associated with provision of second-line treatment. One way to limit the potential financial burden is for the Thai government to make explicit the scope of its commitment to providing public ART: is it a limited commitment to provide only first-line treatment, or is it a more open commitment to provide whatever level of treatment is required by the patient? Estimates of cost-effectiveness show that a version of NAPHA that includes only first-line drugs is much more cost-effective, at only US$736 or B 29,440 per life-year saved, than the policy with second-line therapy. However, NAPHA with second-line therapy saves a quarter of a million more life-years.

A second way for the government to limit its expenditures on second-line therapy is to grant compulsory licenses for the manufacture of patented second-line pharmaceutical products. Doing so will require high-level political resolve that is based on an accurate understanding of the costs to Thailand, the health benefits, the budgetary savings, and the trade repercussions of such action.

Another option would be for the government to explore other financing mechanisms for ART, including greater use of user fees and health insurance schemes. In view of the government's commitment to provide free and universal access to ART through NAPHA, any such plan would have to be carefully designed to avoid excluding people from treatment or discouraging adherence.[5]

Although affordable, expanding ART represents a long-term financial commitment that must be integrated into the budget processes. Once the Thai government begins to finance a patient's AIDS treatment, that access becomes an entitlement that cannot be sacrificed to budget cycles without incurring large political costs. Continuing to support existing ART patients for the rest of their lives and absorbing new ones while maintaining other health programs will require a 24 percent increase in the total health budget by 2013. Because no cure for AIDS is in sight, NAPHA represents a long-term government commitment.

The biggest challenge for Thai health policy makers will be to resist complacency and instead to build a synergistic relationship between treatment and prevention. This approach may require devolution of responsibility for both treatment and prevention to the province level or below so that government units that succeed with prevention will benefit from the saved treatment costs.

Success in rolling out treatment will make achieving the national AIDS strategy objective of less than 1 percent prevalence difficult to attain, because people with HIV will live longer. The first objective of the national AIDS strategy should thus be redefined in terms of HIV incidence, and it should be accompanied by measures to strengthen prevention in the light of expected (and already documented) changes in the risk behavior of both the vulnerable groups and the broader population.

The cost of US$2,145 or B 85,800 per life-year saved through ART may be much more than Thailand would have to spend to save life-years with other interventions. The study recommends that Thailand accompany its expansion of the ART program with vigorous investigation of other promising opportunities to improve health cost-effectively. Prime candidates among those alternatives would be inexpensive HIV prevention programs, including condom distribution and peer education. Expansion of immunization programs, of traffic safety and trauma management, of nutrition programs, and of water supply are all candidates for cost-effective interventions that would save life-years at probably much less than US$2,000 or B 80,000 per year.

## Notes

1. GPO-vir is a single tablet that has a three-drug combination regimen (d4T + 3TC + nevirapine) and is produced by the Government Pharmaceutical Organization (GPO).

2. The details of the AEM and the model assumptions are described in chapter 4.

3. Weights are distributed by 80 percent, 15 percent, and 5 percent, respectively, for the ARV regimes (1), (2), and (3) as shown in table ES.6.

4. These policies to strengthen ART are independent of and much less costly than the decision to finance second-line therapy. They would be even more affordable and advisable if public finance paid only for first-line therapy.

5. Inclusion of AIDS treatment within the "30-Baht" national health care plan, a policy currently under discussion in Thailand, must take into account both the large cost of NAPHA and its uneven geographic distribution across the country. Space constraints prevent an analysis of alternative financing mechanisms for ART in Thailand.

# CHAPTER 1

# Introduction

## International Context and Experience

If left untreated, infection with the human immunodeficiency virus (HIV) is almost universally fatal. Globally, HIV is now the major cause of years of potential life lost and the most common cause of death attributed to an infectious disease. In 2005 alone, 3.1 million people died from AIDS (acquired immunodeficiency syndrome) globally, and 4.9 million people became infected with HIV, bringing to 40.3 million the number of people living with the virus across the world (UNAIDS 2005).

The advent of antiretroviral therapy (ART) in the late 1980s began a revolution in the management of HIV that can be seen as analogous to the use of penicillin for treating bacterial infections in the 1940s. The aim of antiretroviral treatment strategies is suppression of viral replication, and successful treatment leads to immunologic restoration, slowing or halting of disease progression, prevention of drug resistance, and improvement in quality of life. ART is not a cure, but successful use of ART halts the decline in immune deficiency and prevents disease progression and death. ART has radically changed the outlook for those who can pay for it or can use well-resourced health care systems.

Until recently, poor infrastructure and lack of resources were considered major obstacles to the availability of ART in poor countries and among marginal and vulnerable populations. However, growing evidence suggests that provision of ART is both feasible and effective in resource-poor settings. Pilot studies in Africa (Côte d'Ivoire, Kenya, Malawi, Senegal, and Uganda), involving more than 2,000 participants, and one broad-based public health program in Brazil, treating more than 100,000 people, demonstrate the successes of ART:

- significant improvements in weight, CD4 cell count, and viral load
- reductions in the incidence of opportunistic infections
- significant improvements in the quality of life.

Evaluation of the ART program in Brazil in 2002 indicated that during its first seven years 360,000 hospital admissions were avoided, at a savings of US$2.2 billion over the costs of supplying ART; the prevalence of TB was reduced by 80 percent; mortality was reduced by 50 percent; and, following an HIV diagnosis, the median survival increased from 18 months to 58 months (Galvão 2002; Levi and Vitoria 2002). Those results are impressive, and they suggest that it is possible to deliver ART effectively on a large scale in resource-constrained settings.

Of the estimated 40 million adults and children infected with HIV worldwide, at least 5 million to 6 million people would immediately benefit from ART. However, only 700,000 people (approximately 12 percent of the estimated total who urgently need ART) are currently receiving access to therapy on an ongoing basis (WHO 2004a). Thailand, like Brazil, is now at the vanguard of resource-limited countries that are seeking to provide ART as the standard of care to large numbers of people with progressive HIV. As of February 2005, some 52,593 people living with HIV/AIDS (PHAs) in Thailand had received ART through the National Access to Antiretroviral Program for People Living with HIV/AIDS (NAPHA), and approximately 8,000 other PHAs are estimated to have access to ART through the Social Security Scheme (SSS) of the Royal Thai government. The government's objective was to reach a target of 80,000 PHAs by the end of 2005 and a target of 138,000 PHAs by 2007.

## The Hope of ART

The first case of AIDS in Thailand was reported in September 1984. Since then, more than 1 million Thais have been infected with HIV and, of those, more than 400,000 have died. In 2004, some 572,000 Thais were estimated to be living with HIV. Of people living with

HIV, some 50,000 develop serious illness, and a similar number die every year (Thanprasertsuk and others 2004). HIV disease is now the leading cause of premature death in Thailand.

The bulk of this HIV-associated morbidity and mortality falls disproportionately on men and women in their prime productive years: approximately 78 percent of HIV/AIDS cases are in the 25- to 39-year-old group (Thanprasertsuk and others 2004). The human, economic, and social costs of this burden are huge. At the national level, AIDS has reversed the declining trend in national mortality rates, has reduced years of life expectancy, has led to an increase in the number of orphans (expected to reach 200,000 by 2005), and has resulted in sizable losses in labor productivity and years of labor (Phoolcharoen, Posyachinda and others 2004a). At the family level, HIV/AIDS is associated with a high burden of illness, rising medical costs, forgone income, and a need for family members—often elderly parents—to take on the burden of caring for their ill relatives. PHAs also have to confront widespread stigmatization and discrimination, which sometimes extend to their children and families (see box 1.1) (Mohr 2002b).

---

**Box 1.1    Suchada's Story: "ART Is a Great Contribution to Lessen Discrimination"**

When, in 1996, I found out that I was infected, I resigned from my job fearing that people would find out that I was HIV positive. I divorced and moved with my daughter to [an]other province where nobody knew me. We were really alone in this cruel world. It was so hard that I wanted to kill myself, but I could not because I didn't want my child to suffer even more. Four years later, I started to have serious [opportunistic infections] and looked for treatment. Fortunately, I met a doctor who told me about ART and suggested that I should go back to my hometown, where I could join ART free of charge.

It was not easy, because I did not want to disclose myself. I had to contact doctors and nurses privately. Everyone in the community suspected that I was infected. I was discriminated [against], and even my daughter, who is not infected, was discriminated [against]. I could not earn my living, because nobody would buy anything I made to sell in the market. Then I met some PHAs and [nongovernmental organization workers] who gave me good counseling and information. I was encouraged to [im]prove myself. Thanks to ART, my physical appearance is back almost to normal and my health has improved.

I believe that if there were no stigma, no discrimination, HIV/AIDS should be even less serious than many other chronic illnesses. Discrimination is worse than HIV itself. Without discrimination, PHAs are already more than 50 percent "cured." ART is a great contribution to lessen discrimination.

*Source:* Phongphit 2004; personal interviews with PHAs.

---

**Box 1.2   Kamman's Story: The "Miracle" of ART**

I am 29 years old. In 2001, I was diagnos[ed] with HIV. Prior to this, I had been suffering [from] strong headaches, vomiting, and a stiff neck. I also lost weight and started to lose my sight. I left my job and went back home to the northeast. In the provincial hospital, I was advised not to start with [antiretroviral drugs] till I was cured of my OI [opportunistic infection]. In June 2003, I started urinating urine mixed with blood and was advised to go to Khon Kaen University Hospital, where I was told I could start with [antiretroviral drugs]. I had to go to the hospital every week and had to travel a distance of over 200 kilometers and also pay for my [drugs]. Several months later, I was told by a doctor in my province that I could have [medication] also here without paying for it.

It is a surprise and a miracle for many, and also for myself, that with almost all possible OIs, I can still survive and have a life of this quality. My health has improved remarkably since the start of ART six months ago. My weight has increased from 58 kilograms to 75 kilograms, and my CD4 has increased from 0 to 99 [cells per cubic millimeter]. From [being] almost blind, I have recovered part of my sight, and I can now help myself in almost everything and help work at home. Now I can even eat, sleep, and live like ordinary people.

*Source:* Phongphit 2004; personal interviews with PHAs.

---

The Royal Thai government and Thai society have demonstrated a strong commitment to providing comprehensive care and support to PHAs, but only recently have they been able to provide ART to large numbers of people with symptomatic HIV (see chapter 2). The availability of a domestically produced triple-drug combination (GPO-vir) at affordable prices (about B 1,200 or US$30 per month) has opened the door for many PHAs who could previously not afford ART and has allowed the Thai Ministry of Public Health (MOPH) to roll out a large-scale campaign to provide ART in more than 840 hospitals to nearly 52,600 PHAs as of February 2005.[1]

The advent of ART has radically changed the outlook for those living with HIV/AIDS, bringing hope, increased quality of life, reduced stigma, and less discrimination to many PHAs. In the words of an HIV-positive 29-year-old man, ART is a "miracle" (see box 1.2). According to another PHA, with ART she has "recovered my will to live" (see box 1.3). However, as the voices of these PHAs illustrate, using ART is also difficult and painful. As illustrated by box 1.4, many

**Box 1.3  Parichart's Story: "Before ART, I Did Not Want to Live Any Longer"**

I am a widow with a nine-year-old son. I started to take ART in 2001 and initially had to travel a distance of 120 kilometers to Bangkok every month and pay B 5,000. My parents, who are not very well off, had to sell their old car and were also considering selling off a plot of land to buy ART regularly. Now I take ART from the community hospital of my hometown, and I don't have to pay for it.

After [I began] taking ART, my CD4 has increased from 0 to 165 [cells per cubic millimeter], and within six months my weight increased from 42 kilograms to 55 kilograms. I have also been cured of the different OIs (including [tuberculosis], cryptococcal meningitis, [Pneumocystis carinii pneumonia], herpeszoster, etc.) I was suffering with.

Before ART, I did not want to live any longer; now I have recovered my will to live again. I would like to help other PHAs and share my experiences with them. They should know that someone seriously ill, with all kind of OIs like me, can survive. They should have hope, join ART, and take care of their health.

*Source:* Phongphit 2004; personal interviews with PHAs.

PHAs on ART report serious negative side effects and consequences (Phongphit 2004):

- mental and physical side effects

- negative impact on their physical appearance

- drug resistance

- other difficulties.

## Overview of the Report

This report is intended to inform the Royal Thai government and Thai society at large about the full range of benefits, costs, and consequences likely to result from the government's decision to expand public provision of ART through NAPHA and to help design the most effective policies for achieving treatment benefits, promoting prevention, and maintaining financial sustainability.

The report team has structured its analysis around a complex epidemiological model, modified to take into account large-scale provision of ART. This model, the Asian Epidemic Model (AEM), is based

## Box 1.4   Alternatives to ART

### Samran's Story: Drug Resistance

I believe I was infected with HIV in 1987. Four years later, after having lost all hope, I was taken to a temple outside Bangkok, where I received some herbal medicine and gradually regained my health. I went back to Chiang Mai to take other herbal medicine and joined a self-help group of PHAs, where we learned to take care of our health by a "holistic" method, including nutrition, recreation, physical exercise, meditation, herbal medicine, and treatment of OIs.

In 1997, I took AZT and ddI as a member of a trial group. However my health deteriorated. I had OIs on account of drug resistance. After a break of 4 to 5 months, I changed to *Taiomon* from India. In 2001, I started with GPO-vir, and then a [protease inhibitor] group. It did not help, and my health worsened. I had developed drug resistance. Since I stopped ARV, my health is much better. I do not have any OI[s] now, but my CD4 has not gone down below 300 [cells per cubic millimeter], and my viral load is gradually increasing. I have developed drug resistance because I did not have consistency in taking ARV. I think that, although we have ARV, we should not forget to take care of our health holistically.

### Vasna's Story: "If I could go back, I would not join ART"

Ten years ago, while undergoing a voluntary HIV testing and counseling for pregnant women, I found out that I was HIV positive. By January 2003, although I had no OI, I felt tired when walking upstairs, and my CD4 was 100. On [a] doctor's advice, I decided to go on ART.

A year and a month later, I am rather confused about ART. I do not understand why my weight went up from 75 kilograms to 99 kilograms, and I [am] disturbed by the fact that the fat growth is misplaced. If I could go back, I would not join ART till my health would be at its worst point. Because once you take [ART], you have to take the drugs every day of your life without any exception. I would recommend [to] anyone that, as long as his health is still not that bad and [he] has no OI, even if his CD4 is low, he should better take the various alternatives available to keep us healthy before deciding to go for ART. ART should be the last answer to his life.

I think [it] is good that we have ART. Most of my friends and persons I work with and work for have a much better life today thanks to ART. Besides undesired side effects [such] as the ones happening to me, we do not know whether and how long we would have ART, and [if] drug resistance occurs, who could tell us what is next?

*Source:* Phongphit 2004; personal interviews with PHAs.

on available behavioral and transmission data and captures the complexity of HIV risk in Thailand by modeling the behavior of eight separate risk groups. The previous version of this model did not include the effects of ART on the longevity of people with HIV, on their likelihood of transmitting HIV, or on the development and spread of drug-resistant strains of the virus (Thai Working Group on HIV/AIDS Projection 2001). The new version of the AEM, developed for this report, allows for the following factors:

- detailed modeling of early recruitment on the basis of voluntary counseling and treatment (VCT) of asymptomatic patients (at higher CD4 counts) to increasingly substitute for late recruitment of symptomatic patients through the health system (typically at much lower CD4 counts)

- different treatment arms (purely public, augmented public, or private)

- progression into second-line therapy (Brown and Peerapatanapokin 2004a).

Using the AEM, we present the estimated effect of alternative policy scenarios on the following range of indicators that are important to public health and to policy makers:

- reduced numbers of HIV-infected persons

- lengthened lives of HIV-infected people

- reduced costs of hospitalization for opportunistic illnesses

- spread of resistant strains of the virus

- budgetary costs to the government

- both potentially positive and negative effects on prevention activities.

Because the long incubation period of HIV means that the consequences of today's policy choices will play out over decades, all analyses are for a projection period of 25 years. We present the estimated costs and benefits of alternative scenarios and show the sensitivity of the result to the rate at which future costs and benefits are discounted. We draw the model parameters from the Thai literature and experience and, where Thai-specific parameters are not available, from the international

AIDS literature and expert opinion. Sensitivity analysis tests the robustness of the results to alternative assumptions about these parameters.

Because the effect of a policy choice can be defined only in comparison to what would have happened in the absence of that choice, the foundation for the analysis is a baseline projection of the future course of HIV/AIDS treatment if the Royal Thai government had neither introduced its expanded NAPHA nor subsidized the production and sales of low-cost generic ART (GPO-vir) through the Government Pharmaceutical Organization (GPO). In other words, the baseline scenario assumes no significant public role in the provision or financing of ART, or it assumes a very limited role, such as the MOPH's previously existing, very small, voluntary program, which operated through the clinical research network and reached only some 2,100 people.[2] Although alternative baseline scenarios could have been chosen, the report team deemed this baseline to be the cleanest and simplest to interpret (see chapter 4 for the details of the baseline).

Against this baseline projection, we analyze the effect of the government's NAPHA under several alternative versions of its implementation. The policy options considered for NAPHA explore, on the one hand, ways to facilitate earlier recruitment into ART by strengthening and stimulating demand for VCT for HIV and, on the other hand, ways to encourage adherence through PHA groups, use of counselors, conditional transfers, and other demand-side programs.[3] This range of policy options for NAPHA is summarized in table 1.1.

**Table 1.1**  Policy Scenarios for NAPHA

| | | Encourage VCT and early recruitment into ART | |
|---|---|---|---|
| | | No | Yes |
| Encourage adherence through demand-side incentives such as PHA groups, accompagnateurs, and conditional transfers | No | NAPHA (D1): Current implementation of NAPHA (recruit mainly symptomatic HIV-infected persons through the public health system) | VCT (D2): Earlier recruitment through VCT of people with higher CD4 counts, without improved adherence |
| | Yes | Adherence (D3): Improved adherence without earlier recruitment (keep current recruitment of symptomatic HIV-infected persons through the public health system) | VCT and adherence (D4): Improved adherence and earlier recruitment (recruit earlier through VCT of people with higher CD4 counts) |

Source: Author.

We compute the projected HIV epidemic under each of these scenarios, and then we estimate the effect of each scenario on the range of key indicators described above. Indicator outcomes under these scenarios are compared against the baseline of no ART, as discussed earlier. We then compute cost-effectiveness measures of the alternative policy options.

The report is organized into seven chapters. Chapter 2 describes the dynamics and patterns of the HIV epidemic in Thailand and summarizes the Thai policy response. Chapter 3 presents a brief technical discussion of the clinical management of HIV/AIDS, including challenges faced in the clinical management of ART; its effect on survival, infectivity, and transmission; and its socioeconomic effect. Chapter 3 also synthesizes the information available on the costs associated with ART—treatment of opportunistic infections and VCT—to both the household and the public health care system. That information is then used to estimate the costs and benefits of ART under different scenarios. Chapter 4 presents an analytical framework for the evaluation of ART treatment policy and presents the estimated effect of current NAPHA policy on such treatment. The framework computes the cost-effectiveness of current policy and discusses its fiscal and financial implications. Chapter 5 expands this analysis by evaluating the costs and benefits of the alternative policy scenarios (see table 1.1 for scenarios D2–D4). Chapter 6 carries out some sensitivity analyses on key biological and behavioral parameters and on assumptions about the evolution of prices for second-line therapy. Finally, chapter 7 concludes and presents the team's recommendations. Technical details and data are synthesized in the annexes.

## Notes

1. See NAPHA website from the Bureau of AIDS. TB, and STI at MOPH (2005) for the PHA figures: http://www.aidsthai.org/care. The figure on PHAs cited is accessible on this website.

2. See chapter 2 and the background papers by Gold and others (2005) and Thanprasertsuk and others (2005) for a detailed description of the evolution of the government's ART program.

3. For example, by using paid adherence counselors with little medical training (accompagnateurs), the Partners in Health program in Haiti has had substantial adherence (Farmer and others, 2001a, 2001b, 2003).

# The Thai AIDS Epidemic Now

## The Epidemiology of HIV in the Thai Population

Although every country's AIDS epidemic is unique, Thailand's epidemic stands out both for the complexity of its epidemiological history and for the vigor of the government's response.

### Trends and Transmission of the Epidemic over Time

The dynamics of the Thai epidemic have been well documented in numerous studies, including those by Brown and others (1994); Phoolcharoen and others (1998); Weniger and others (1991) and the World Bank (1997, 1999, 2000). Nevertheless, it is useful to revisit briefly some of its main features.

The first cases of AIDS in Thailand were reported in 1984. Progressive numbers of AIDS cases and HIV infections were reported throughout the following years as the epidemic spread in a series of waves in subgroups of the population identified by all the major transmission routes: homosexuals, injecting drug users (IDUs), heterosexuals, and mothers of newborns (World Bank 2000). Between 1984 and 1987, cases were largely confined to homosexual male Thais. This period was followed by an explosive spread of HIV infection among IDUs in 1987 and 1988, when prevalence rates among IDUs in Bangkok jumped from virtually 0 to 40 percent (MOPH 2002b). The virus then spread to sex workers and their clients in 1989 and 1990, with the result that heterosexual transmission became an increasingly important route. By 1994, HIV prevalence[1]—the percentage of the population currently infected—had reached 31 percent nationally among brothel-based sex workers and 38 percent in the northern region of Thailand (MOPH 2002b). Use of commercial sex was widespread: a national behavioral survey in 1990 found that 22 percent of men ages 15 to 49, and 37 percent of men ages 20 to 24 had visited a sex worker in the past year (Sittitrai 1992). Condom use in commercial sex was quite low—only 38 percent of men who frequently used sex workers in the 1990 study used condoms all the time. Accordingly, HIV spread rapidly between sex workers and their clients. By 1994, 1 in 10 clients was infected with the virus. Those clients then infected their wives, who in turn became pregnant and transmitted HIV to their children. In 1991, the first perinatal cases were reported, and the numbers of infected newborns increased in the following years.

The trend of the epidemic is charted in figure 2.1, which presents prevalence rates for pregnant women and 21-year-old male conscripts for the 1989–2003 period. HIV prevalence among young male conscripts peaked in 1993 at 4 percent nationally (and at nearly 13 percent in the north), but it has since come down sharply (World Bank 2000). The same pattern is observed for prevalence rates among sex workers (figure 2.2). HIV prevalence rates among women attending prenatal clinics (a low-risk group) follow the same pattern, but with a lag, rising from about 0.89 percent in 1989 to 2.3 percent in 1995,

**Figure 2.1** HIV Prevalence among Pregnant Women, Blood Donors, and 21-Year-Old Male Conscripts

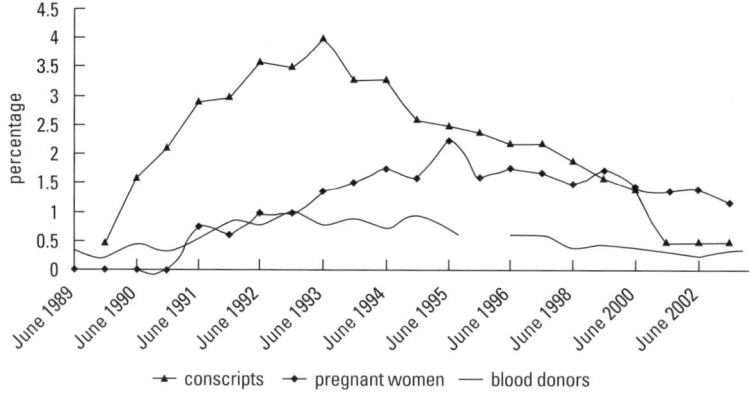

*Source:* MOPH 2004; Thanprasertsuk 2004.

**Figure 2.2** HIV Prevalence among Direct and Indirect Sex Workers

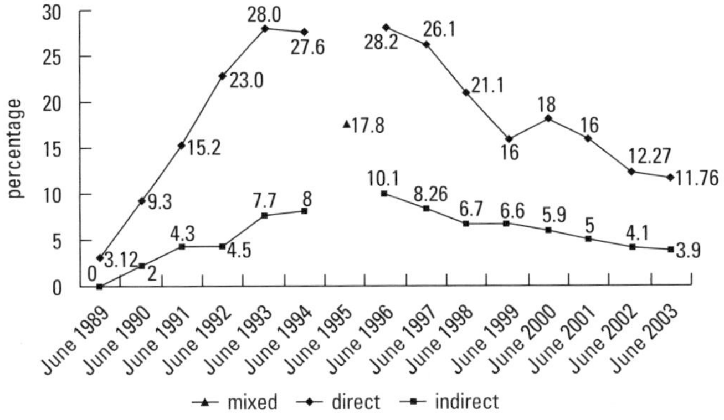

*Source:* MOPH 2004; Thanprasertsuk 2004.

before starting to come down. A comparison of figures 2.1 and 2.2 reveals that the prevalence rate among the high-risk groups of sex workers and their clients (as proxied by young male conscripts) was an accurate leading indicator of the prevalence rate among low-risk groups and the general population. This finding suggests that sentinel surveillance of high-risk groups can help policy makers anticipate changes in the general epidemic.

Although HIV prevalence rates have come down dramatically since the mid-1990s, the HIV/AIDS crisis in Thailand is far from over. The last waves of new infections among women and their children have only recently started to decline, and prevalence rates among certain at-risk groups remain very high. Prevalence rates among IDUs—the group with the highest prevalence—are still close to 50 percent and have not declined since the late 1990s (figure 2.3). Prevalence rates among commercial sex workers declined considerably in response to Thailand's strong national response and the 100 percent condom program. Nevertheless, sex workers remain a major risk group. In 2003, the prevalence rate was 11.7 percent among female direct sex workers and 3.9 percent among indirect sex workers. Other high-prevalence groups include male sex workers (7.9 percent), fishermen (6.9 percent), and males presenting at clinics with sexually transmitted infections (STIs) (4.6 percent) (Thanprasertsuk 2004). With a large number of people infected with HIV, the potential for the epidemic to spread if prevention efforts are relaxed is considerable.

**Figure 2.3** HIV Prevalence among IDUs

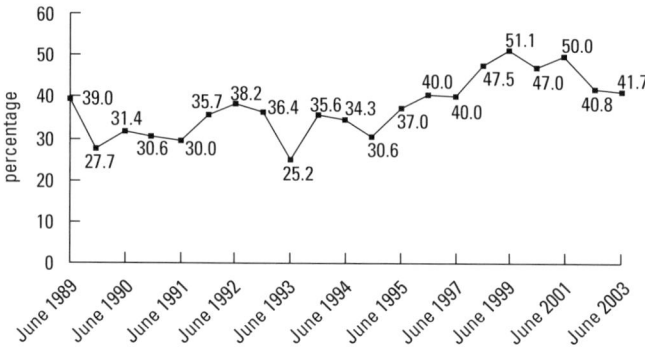

*Source:* MOPH 2004; Thanprasertsuk 2004.

In 2001, the Thai Working Group on HIV/AIDS projected that by 2004 about 572,500 Thais would be living with HIV/AIDS (table 2.1). Among them, approximately 49,500 would develop serious AIDS-related illnesses in 2004, and about the same number would die of AIDS-related complications. The group also estimated that 19,500 new HIV infections would occur in 2004 (compared with 143,000 new infections in 1990 and 23,676 new infections in 2002).

Almost 80 percent of all AIDS cases will occur among people ages 20 to 39. Heterosexual transmission remains the main mode of transmission, accounting for the bulk of all AIDS cases. But the composition of infections has changed dramatically. A decade ago, most of the infections were in adults, and 80 percent were in sex workers and their clients. Now about one-half of all new infections are in women infected by their husbands or sex partners. IDUs account for about 5 percent of reported infections. Approximately 4 percent of AIDS cases in Thailand occur in children, and in 2000, one-seventh of new infections were in children.

**Table 2.1** Estimated Cumulative Numbers for HIV/AIDS, 2004

| Statistic | Number |
|---|---|
| Total HIV infections (adults and children) up to 2004 | 1,074,155 |
| Total cumulative deaths (adults and children) up to 2004 | 501,600 |
| People living with HIV in 2004 | 572,484 |
| Projected new HIV infections in 2004 | 19,471 |
| Projected new AIDS cases in 2004 | 49,542 |

*Source:* Thai Working Group on HIV/AIDS Projection 2001.

**Figure 2.4**   Projected Annual New AIDS Cases

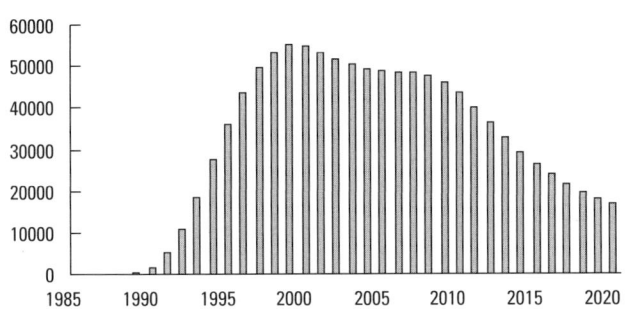

*Source:* Thai Working Group Projection 2001.

The demand for HIV/AIDS treatment and care is rising as Thailand's epidemic enters a new phase, with many of those infected during the early years of the epidemic becoming ill with symptomatic disease.[2] The current number of new annual AIDS cases—just under 50,000—is projected to remain constant until 2006, when it should start to decline because of the sharp reduction in new infections in the late 1990s (figure 2.4). Meeting this demand for care poses a huge challenge to the Royal Thai government and Thai society. In a few years, as AIDS patients live longer with antiretroviral therapy (ART), the health system will need to provide care not only to 10,000 to 20,000 new cases per year but also to many of those whose lives have been significantly prolonged by ART.

The National Access to Antiretrovirals Program for People Living with HIV/AIDS (NAPHA) is a comprehensive and ambitious attempt to provide such care, with ART as the standard. By all measures, given the commitment across all segments of Thai society, the country's significant health system capacity, and the availability of internal and external financing, Thailand has a strong chance of meeting this challenge. But its ability to even contemplate providing care to all those who need it rests on the success of its past national prevention efforts.

Without those efforts, HIV infections—and hence AIDS cases—would be as much as 14 times higher than they are today (figure 2.5) (Thai Working Group on HIV/AIDS Projection 2001). We estimate that, without such efforts, Thailand would have had 7.7 million HIV cases and 850,000 AIDS cases in 2005, roughly 14 times more of each than was the case. If Thailand were to try to offer ART to this much larger number of AIDS patients, its budget requirements would also be 14 times greater—and they would continue to grow over the next

**Figure 2.5** Projected HIV Infections in the Absence of Successful Prevention Effort

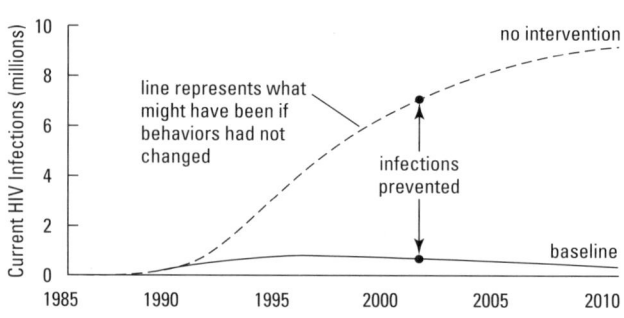

*Source:* Thai Working Group on HIV/AIDS Projection 2001.

decade. Thanks to its substantial prevention efforts from 1991 to 2002, Thailand has avoided the need to spend an additional US$18.6 billion (B 745 billion) on treatment over the decade through 2012.

During the 1990s, Thailand spent more than most countries on its HIV/AIDS program. Its total budget expenditure on prevention and treatment combined over this period was a substantial US$434 million in 2002 dollars (B 17.3 billion). However, by averting the need to spend US$18.6 billion (B 745 billion) over the subsequent decade, the government saved US$43 (or B 1720) for each dollar (or baht) invested in the 1990s. It is doubtful that any other Thai government investment achieved such a high benefit-cost ratio.

This experience offers a critical lesson for other countries about the importance of prevention. When the finance ministries of such countries as China and India—where the HIV/AIDS epidemic is at an earlier stage—make intersectoral allocations of the government's budget, they should be aware of the high return to HIV/AIDS prevention campaigns. The experience also offers an essential lesson to Thai policy makers on the importance of not allowing the demand for treatment and care to crowd out continued prevention efforts.

### Spatial Patterns of HIV/AIDS in Thailand

The HIV epidemic in Thailand presents some distinct spatial and geographic patterns, which lead to very different needs across regions and geographic areas in terms of availability of treatment. The epidemic started in the northern region, and this region still contains the largest number of people living with HIV/AIDS (PHAs), as well as the largest number of people who are symptomatic and in need of treatment. But since the start of the epidemic, HIV has spread to all other regions of Thailand. As the number of new infections has come down in the north—the result of aggressive and successful prevention efforts among the main risk groups—it has risen in other regions. Infections among IDUs and indirect sex workers have been rising in Bangkok, the central region, and the south.

The latest figures from the 21st round of the seroprevalence surveys shows prevalence rates for IDUs in the central and southern regions of about 50 percent. In Bangkok, HIV prevalence rates among direct sex workers rose between 1996 and 2000. Although prevalence rates among male conscripts have declined across most regions, the decline has been much sharper in the upper north than in other areas. In the south, the prevalence rate among male conscripts (a proxy for the prevalence of HIV in the general male population) has stagnated at a relatively high level of 2.4 percent. It actually increased slightly in Bangkok between 1993 and 2000 (World Bank 2000). Prevalence rates among male clients of sexually transmitted infection (STI) clinics are much higher in the central and southern regions (at 6.9 percent and 7.5 percent, respectively) than the national rate for the same group (4 percent).

Map 2.1, located in the Map section at the end of the book, shows the spatial distribution of cumulative AIDS cases in Thailand by province for 1986 to 2003 and the spatial distribution of symptomatic HIV cases reported through the public health system as of March 2004. Map 2.2 presents the same two variables at the district (*amphoe*) level. Both maps illustrate the spatial patterns of the epidemic in Thailand, showing a high concentration of both reported AIDS cases and symptomatic HIV cases in the north (with particular concentration in some districts) and in Bangkok—where people were infected earlier and are at a more advanced stage of disease. Nevertheless, both AIDS and symptomatic cases are reported in all parts of Thailand. Over time, as many of those infected later become symptomatic, the concentration of cases in the central and southern regions will increase. It is interesting to note that almost all provinces have pockets (districts) with high prevalence rates of AIDS or symptomatic HIV.

Although a substantial literature exists on the dynamics of HIV transmission in Thailand, empirical research on the socioeconomic determinants of HIV infection is quite scarce.[3] In bivariate analyses, the numbers of HIV or AIDS cases in a province or district are not strongly associated with indices of poverty or inequality.

Multivariate analysis of the determinants of HIV infection, allowing for spatial correlation across neighboring geographic units, is under way (Beegle and others 2006).

## Policy Response to the Epidemic

Thailand is now widely recognized for its progressive policy response to HIV/AIDS, but this was not always the case.[4] Initially the policy response was muted. Only when HIV infections exploded among IDUs and sex workers in 1988 and 1989 did the government respond and act decisively with a nationwide, multisectoral HIV/AIDS prevention campaign. The campaign was hugely successful in changing behavior and lowering the rate of new infection among commercial sex workers and their clients. Since then, the national policy response has evolved, driven by the changing nature and stage of the HIV/AIDS epidemic and by innovation and progress in instruments of both prevention and treatment. Throughout, policies and programs have been strongly influenced both by epidemiological, social, and behavioral data and, very significantly, by the efforts of PHA networks, PHA activists, and the nongovernmental organization (NGO) community (Phoolcharoen and others 2004b; Thanprasertsuk and others 2004; World Bank 2000).

Thailand's success in lowering HIV incidence rates and combating the epidemic, however, leaves no room for complacency. Some of the riskiest behaviors in Thailand (among IDUs, men having sex with men, and indirect sex workers) have not been fully addressed and stand out as major causes of continued HIV transmission (World Bank 2000). Moreover, as the demand for HIV/AIDS-related medical care and treatment grows, so does the risk that prevention efforts will be relaxed and Thailand's success in controlling the epidemic jeopardized.

### The Three Phases of the National Response

#### Phase 1: Public Health–Focused Phase
In the early years of the epidemic, policy largely followed a focused public health approach to HIV control. The government response was confined mainly to the Ministry of Public Health (MOPH), which established a case reporting system that required all health settings in

the country to report possible cases to its newly established AIDS Control Center. This system failed to detect the rapid spread of HIV infection, which is asymptomatic for many years before it progresses to AIDS. Between 1984 and 1989, only 43 AIDS cases and 145 AIDS-related complex cases were reported, even though subsequent reconstruction of the dynamics of the epidemic showed that more than 100,000 HIV infections had occurred by 1989 (Phoolcharoen and others 1998). At that stage, no surveillance surveys had been done, and small surveys of seroprevalence in Bangkok through 1987 found little evidence of HIV. Information on the extent of risky behavior that might spread HIV in the general population was very limited.

The first evidence that HIV could spread rapidly in the Thai population did not appear until 1988, when HIV testing was introduced in government methadone treatment centers for heroin addicts, revealing very high rates of prevalence (Phoolcharoen and others 2004a). This finding coincided with cabinet approval of the Medium-Term Program for the Prevention and Control of AIDS, 1989–91. This program was intended to provide a working framework for government, NGO, and private initiatives, including measures for program management, health education, counseling, training, surveillance, monitoring, medical and social care, and laboratory and blood safety control. However, most funding for HIV/AIDS activities through 1990 came from external sources, including international organizations and bilateral aid. Internal resource mobilization was very limited (Phoolcharoen and others 2004a; Thanprasertsuk and others 2004b; World Bank 2000).

The explosive spread of HIV among IDUs prompted the Royal Thai Army and the Epidemiology Division of MOPH to launch a national HIV surveillance survey of key population groups in 1989. Testing was launched in samples of 100 to 200 persons from each of several sentinel groups—IDUs, brothel-based sex workers, male sex workers, male patients at STI clinics, blood donors, pregnant women, new prisoners, and ex-prisoners. Testing began in 14 provinces and was expanded to all 73 provinces by 1990.[5] Simultaneously, the army launched biannual testing of the 60,000 21-year old army conscripts chosen annually by national lottery, finding an HIV prevalence of 0.5 percent during the first round. Since then, the prevalence of HIV among Thai conscripts has been used as a surrogate marker of infection in young Thai males. The first national survey of behavioral risks for HIV infection (the Partner Relations Survey) was launched in 1990, sponsored by the World Health Organization (WHO) and conducted by the Thai Red Cross and Chulalongkorn University. The systematic and periodic Behavioral Surveillance Survey (BSS) was started in 1995.

Early on, policies were put in place to ensure that the nation's blood supply was protected. Nevertheless, the government downplayed the significance of the epidemic to the general population. It did little to correct the perception that HIV was likely to affect only marginal groups such as gay men, male sex workers, and IDUs and focused its preventive concerns on those groups (World Bank 2000). In 1989, prominent activists inside and outside government lent their credibility and prestige to the anti-AIDS campaign. Armed with the findings of the first round of sentinel surveillance and joined by a growing number of NGOs concerned about human rights and the spread of HIV in their communities, these activists were able to raise awareness and initiate the process of change. By 1990, the administration was showing signs of increasing recognition that HIV/AIDS prevention and control needed to be a government and development priority. In January 1990, Prime Minister Chatichai Choonhavan announced an official campaign to prevent and control HIV/AIDS. This announcement was the first clear-cut government stance on AIDS (Phoolcharoen and others 2004a; Thanprasertsuk and others 2004; World Bank 2000).

*Phase 2: Socially Focused and Multisectoral Phase (1991–96)*
In 1991, under the brief government of Prime Minister Anand Panyarachun (1991–92), AIDS prevention and control became a national priority at the highest level. AIDS policy was brought under the coordination of the Office of the Prime Minister, with the establishment of an official multisectoral National AIDS Prevention and Control Committee, chaired by the prime minister. This move signaled commitment at the highest political level and also allowed for the formal participation of NGOs in the policy-making process. The National Economic and Social Development Board (NESDB) was given responsibility for planning the national AIDS strategy. The result was the first five-year AIDS control program and budget, which allocated funds to a number of government agencies and NGOs. The plan emphasized mobilizing society and communities to participate in the prevention of HIV, to care for those who are sick, and to reduce stigma and discrimination (World Bank 2000). This type of strategic, multisectoral HIV/AIDS plan has continued to be formulated and implemented.

A massive public information campaign on AIDS was launched under the leadership of a highly respected Thai figure, Mechai Viravaidya, through the mass media. The messages emphasized prevention, behavior change, and condom use and identified AIDS as a social problem, not just a health problem. All ministries were recruited to actively educate and train their staffs, and the Ministry of Education was asked to launch peer education groups. Private initiatives by business and NGOs complemented the government's efforts.

The 100 Percent Condom Program was adopted nationwide to promote universal use of condoms in commercial sex all the time. The mechanisms for monitoring compliance already existed through Thailand's extensive network of STI clinics. Under the program, sex workers were screened for STIs weekly or biweekly at government STI clinics, were treated, and then were provided with a box of 100 free condoms (World Bank 2000). The presentation of male patients at STI clinics was considered evidence of lack of use of condoms, and the sources were traced back to the brothels where the men were infected. Health workers then followed up with visits to the brothels, during which they provided information and condoms.

The campaign was very effective: condom use among direct sex workers went from 14 percent at the start of the program to nearly 100 percent. Recent sentinel surveys suggest that condom use among direct sex workers remains high (although not universal) at about 95 percent (figure 2.6). The campaign had somewhat less success among

**Figure 2.6**  Condom Use among Commercial Sex Workers

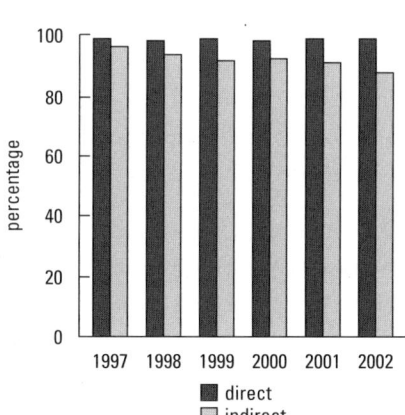

*Source:* MOPH 2004; Thanprasertsuk 2004.

indirect sex workers. In a worrisome trend, condom use among indirect sex workers may have recently declined to as low as 85 percent (Thanprasertsuk 2004). MOPH officials acknowledge that such a decline in condom use among indirect sex workers is a cause for concern and signals the need to relaunch the campaign to encourage more condom use among all sex workers.

Since the start of the campaign, condom promotion has been extended to target a broader array of risk groups, with mixed success. As shown in figure 2.6, condom use is not universal among indirect sex workers; it is even lower among male sex workers—a group not originally targeted by the 100 Percent Condom Program. In a Chiang Mai survey, just over 50 percent of male sex workers reported consistent condom use with clients; consistent use with noncommercial partners was markedly lower. Other groups in which condom use is likely to be low are illegal or undocumented sex workers (many of them migrants from the Lao People's Democratic Republic, Myanmar, and other neighboring countries) and migrant fishermen from Cambodia and Myanmar.

Inconsistent condom use among the general public is another major gap in the population's defenses against HIV. Behavioral Surveillance Surveys in the past five years suggest that risky sexual behavior patterns have shifted away from men visiting sex workers to men having sexual relationships with casual female partners or girlfriends, and with other men (Thanprasertsuk 2004). The rate of condom use in these other types of relationships (including those with casual female partners or steady girlfriends) is quite low. The most recent round of the BSS among military conscripts reports a rate of condom use in first sexual experiences of 22.6 percent. Consistent condom use with female sex workers is reported by only 59 percent of respondents, and only 25 percent of respondents report consistent condom use with irregular female partners.

*Phase 3: The Holistic Phase (1997 to present)*
The growing number of AIDS cases (including those among children) and the increasing awareness of the extent of HIV infection in the Thai population gradually built a national understanding that no community would remain unaffected. This realization happened at the same time that the NESDB planning efforts were moving in directions strongly focused on building the capacity of all communi-

ties to participate in the overall development process. These forces combined to move the Thai response to HIV/AIDS in new directions. In 1995, the NESDB was entrusted with the formulation of a new national AIDS strategic plan for 1997 to 2001. The planning process was a participatory one, involving a wide spectrum of agencies across sectors as well as networks of PHAs. This process took advantage of the experience in HIV/AIDS prevention and care gained in the first decade of the Thai epidemic. The resulting program gave PHAs an important role as an essential human resource in the fight against HIV/AIDS. Collaboration between PHA groups and between PHA networks and the national program was enhanced to allow PHAs to become active partners in planning and implementing a wide range of HIV/AIDS programs from the national level to community levels.

Building on experience, the plan provided for a number of specific strategies to strengthen the HIV/AIDS policy response:

• continued awareness campaigns

• reinforcement of traditional community support networks

• integration of life skills training into school curricula

• expansion of health promotion activities and medical care for those with HIV/AIDS in both public health and community settings.

The key objective was to establish mechanisms to deliver health and welfare services to PHAs in a holistic manner, covering prevention, care, and alleviation of the socioeconomic impact of AIDS.

*National Plan for the Prevention and Alleviation of HIV/AIDS (2002–6)*
The most recent HIV/AIDS plan is in actuality a continuation of the previous plan, sharing the same holistic approach and emphasis on the participation of private and public sectors, as well as communities, in the fight against AIDS. This plan sets forth three targets:

• HIV prevalence rates among the reproductive-age population to be reduced to less than 1 percent by 2006

• at least 80 percent of PHAs and affected individuals to have access to and be receiving care and support from public, private, and community providers of social, economic, educational, and primary health care services in an appropriate and fair manner

- local administrations and community organizations to be efficiently and continuously planning and carrying out plans for HIV/AIDS prevention and alleviation.

Some of the main strategies of the national plan include

- Promotion of condom use and sex education among youth.

- Prevention of mother-to-child transmission (PMTCT) of HIV. Voluntary counseling and testing (VCT) for pregnant women was introduced in 1995 and has been gradually expanded to reach 559,702 women in 2002. About 1.1 percent were found to be HIV positive. Among these, 80 percent received a short regimen of AZT (zidovudine) during the prenatal period and delivery, as did 95 percent of infants born to HIV-positive mothers. In 2003, the regimen for PMTCT was revised to include AZT plus nevirapine. The effect has been to reduce the risk of transmission to the child from 30 percent to 8 percent, resulting in the aversion of 2,500 to 3,000 child infections each year.

- VCT. Counseling and testing is available at nearly all provincial and district hospitals, at selected health centers, and through the private sector.

- Reduction of transmission among IDUs. Drug treatment programs have been initiated in Bangkok and five regional drug treatment centers.

- Access to care (subsequently expanded into NAPHA). Services for treatment and prophylaxis of common opportunistic infections are being expanded to ensure coverage. Services are also being developed to provide combination ART for all symptomatic HIV-positive individuals, with a target to reach all estimated 80,000 HIV-positive people by the end of 2005.

- Community responses. Measures have been taken to promote community role in organizing and implementing prevention, care, and support activities, especially in rural areas.

- Support to networks of NGOs and PHAs. The Thai NGO Coalition on AIDS represents more than 300 NGOs working on AIDS throughout Thailand, and the Thai Network of People Living with HIV has a network of more than 300 PHA organizations throughout the country. Both are represented on the National AIDS Committee.

*Impact, Lessons Learned, and Risks*

The success of Thailand's strong national policy response to HIV/AIDS has been extensively documented (Chamratrithirong and others 1999; Phoolcharoen and others 1998; Phoolcharoen and others 2004a; World Bank 2000). The Thai experience is often evoked as an example of how a national response that effectively mobilizes government, NGOs, and the private sector can be effective in controlling a growing epidemic through relatively simple interventions.

A number of factors worked in Thailand's favor:

• political commitment at the highest level

• the ability to draw on strong institutions, including an established network of STI clinics, a successful family planning program, a cadre of trained epidemiologists, and health infrastructure with qualified staff

• a strong civil society with a tradition of activism and volunteerism

• an established network of NGOs.

However, Thailand's successful response also required a significant commitment of national resources. Starting in 1990, the Thai government devoted a large amount of its budget to its AIDS program. Between 1987 and 1997, public spending on AIDS prevention and control in Thailand expanded dramatically to reach some US$82 million annually by 1997. As much as 96 percent of this was financed by the Thai government. This amount was equivalent to about one-fourth of the entire international expenditure on AIDS programs in the developing world at the time (World Bank 1999).

Thailand's successful prevention interventions had a large effect on the course of the epidemic. Recent estimates from the Asian Epidemic Model (AEM), suggest that, in the absence of these interventions, the current number of infections would be nearly 14 times higher than the number we observe today. As shown in figure 2.5, almost 7.7 million people would be infected. There is no room for complacency, however. Although policies successfully lowered prevalence rates, a large number of Thais were infected with HIV in the early years, when the epidemic took hold in the population. As a result, more than 1 million Thais have been infected with HIV and more than 400,000 have died. Estimates suggest that more than 572,000 people are currently infected with HIV in 2004 and that nearly 50,000 of them will develop AIDS. Providing care and treatment for these large numbers of people presents a challenge to the public health system. Moreover, the prevalence of HIV in high-risk groups is still high—especially among groups that were not explicitly targeted by prevention efforts in the past, such as IDUs or male sex workers. The prevalence rate among IDUs remains very high (in excess of 40 percent) and has not come down.

Evidence also exists that the effect of past prevention campaigns is waning. Recent rounds of the BSS show that the percentage of male conscripts reporting sexual relationships with commercial sex workers, after declining for several years, started to pick up again in 2002 and 2003. The same pattern is visible with the percentages of male conscripts reporting other female sex partners and of married conscripts who have extramarital sex. Condom use among these male conscripts is not high: only 59 percent report consistent use of condoms with sex workers, and only 25 percent do so with irregular female sex partners. New risk behaviors by other groups of the population, such as youth (box 2.1), also need to be addressed. In 2002 and 2003, the BSS found a sharp increase in the proportion of grade 11 students who report having sexual relationships with girlfriends or boyfriends. Among grade 11 male students, there was also a rebound in the proportion who have sexual relationships with commercial sex workers. Prevention efforts targeted at these groups need to be strengthened and to be extended to the general population.

## Thailand's ART Program

A discussion of Thailand's ART program must begin with a description of past measures of ART provision.[6]

### Past Provision of ART in Thailand
Figure 2.7 shows the progression of HIV/AIDS treatment in Thailand. Several phases were involved.

**Phase 1: Introduction of ART** Thailand commenced publicly funded ART in 1992. The MOPH's priority at the time was provision of a single-drug treatment (AZT monotherapy) to low-income groups. Only a handful of referral and university hospitals participated in the program. Because of the high cost of the drugs, the initial budget of B 35 million (US$875,000) increased to B 300 million (US$7.5 million)

## Box 2.1 Youth and HIV/AIDS in Thailand

*Hardly a taboo now, sex among youths is a fact of life as Thai attitudes about sex have become more open, especially among young people.*

—"Don't Leave Love Out of All the Sex Talk," *Nation,* February 14, 2004

A shift of mindset is required in order to work on youth HIV/AIDS issues in Thailand. What proved successful in the old days may not work as well in the current environment. The dynamics of the epidemic of HIV/AIDS in Thailand are changing. Spreading patterns are now not limited to the traditionally defined risk groups. Young people are emerging as a new group at risk: not only are they having sex at a younger age than before, but they also have a very low condom usage rate. Recently, the MOPH conducted a survey among public school male students in grade 11 (15 to 20 years old) in 20 provinces, covering the period 1996–2003. The surveys were conducted in seven rounds (one each year), with an average sample of 5,440 per round. In 1996, the survey found that 9.8 percent of male students had had their first sexual relationship by grade 11; this figure had risen to 13.2 percent by 2003. The survey also showed very low rates of condom use among male students, especially in relationships with their girlfriends or close friends (only 9.4 to 17.5 percent reported using condoms). In the case of male students who had sex with men, the condom usage rate was not much better: 3.9 to 25 percent.

Accepting changing sexual behavior among youth requires a significant shift in entrenched conservative mores and attitudes in Thai society. The MOPH has been spearheading a strong prevention campaign aimed at youth, but many of the measures—such as the introduction of condom vending machines in universities—have met substantial resistance. The MOPH's prevention efforts need greater support from other ministries and from society at large. A top priority is achieving greater cooperation with (and stronger support from) the Ministry of Education to include life skills in the curriculum, to provide access to information about HIV, and to disseminate basic knowledge about the disease through the school system. Other government initiatives related to youth and their sexual behavior include

- a proposal for a youth curfew
- introduction of a program to block access to Web sites with gambling or pornographic content
- other public relations activities to dissuade teenagers from having sex when they are not "ready," such as providing AIDS information sessions in schools and regulating academic dormitories.

**Figure 2.7** Access to HIV/AIDS Medical Care

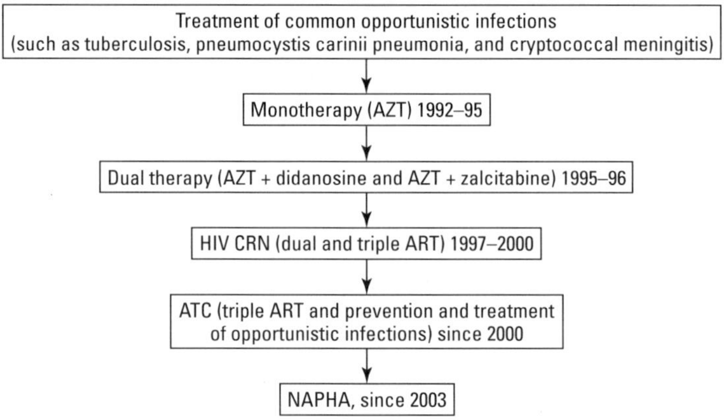

```
┌─────────────────────────────────────────────────────────────────────────┐
│                 Treatment of common opportunistic infections              │
│ (such as tuberculosis, pneumocystis carinii pneumonia, and cryptococcal meningitis) │
└─────────────────────────────────────────────────────────────────────────┘
                                    ↓
                    ┌───────────────────────────────┐
                    │  Monotherapy (AZT) 1992–95    │
                    └───────────────────────────────┘
                                    ↓
          ┌──────────────────────────────────────────────────────┐
          │ Dual therapy (AZT + didanosine and AZT + zalcitabine) 1995–96 │
          └──────────────────────────────────────────────────────┘
                                    ↓
                ┌────────────────────────────────────────┐
                │ HIV CRN (dual and triple ART) 1997–2000 │
                └────────────────────────────────────────┘
                                    ↓
              ┌──────────────────────────────────────────┐
              │ ATC (triple ART and prevention and treatment │
              │   of opportunistic infections) since 2000  │
              └──────────────────────────────────────────┘
                                    ↓
                       ┌──────────────────────┐
                       │  NAPHA, since 2003   │
                       └──────────────────────┘
```

*Source:* MOPH 2004; Thanprasertsuk 2004.

by 1997, yet the number of patients enrolled in the program was low. An economic review of this antiretroviral supply program, carried out by the World Bank, WHO, and MOPH in 1995, concluded that it demonstrated high cost and low benefit to the targeted population (Kunanusont and others 1995). This conclusion was based on the low coverage rate, poor patient adherence, and high rates of loss to follow-up (Prescott 1997).

*Phase 2: Clinical Research Network*   Following this review, the focus of the ART program was switched. Instead of the MOPH acting as a central supply of antiretrovirals to its hospitals, a clinical research network (CRN) distributed antiretroviral drugs to selected hospitals that agreed to participate in operational research. This link of clinical research to access to comprehensive care, including antiretroviral drugs, for patients with HIV/AIDS continued to be the basis of the publicly funded antiretroviral program until 2000. The program formed part of the National Strategy for the Prevention and Treatment of HIV/AIDS, which included programs for PMTCT, a safe donated blood supply, and HIV vaccine development, as well as the condom use campaign. The network initially consisted of 45 hospitals (expanded to 58) in 20 provinces and provided ART to 1,095 patients. Monotherapy was initially used, but starting in 1998, dual therapy with an appropriate combination of antiretroviral drugs became the standard treatment.

The effect of the CRN was evaluated in July 2000. A report commissioned by the WHO in collaboration with the Division of AIDS,

Department of Communicable Diseases, MOPH, was published on December 21, 2000 (MOPH 2000). The report concluded that, during the three years of operation of the CRN, its effect on program planning for HIV/AIDS prevention and care was limited because its roles in clinical research and prevention and care activities were not clearly defined, the hospitals and research institutions in the network had too many tasks, and the network was underresourced.

***Phase 3: Move Toward National Access to ART***   In 2000, the MOPH established a pilot Access to Care (ATC) initiative to provide ART through the CRN and an additional 109 district and provincial hospitals, expanding access to another 1,000 patients. Criteria for enrollment into the program were

- having been diagnosed with an AIDS-defining opportunistic infection or cancer

- having symptomatic HIV

- having a CD4 count of less than 200 cells per cubic millimeter.

The initiative offered 8 ART regimens for adults and 12 regimens for children. About 78 percent of patients received two nucleoside reverse transcriptase inhibitors (NRTIs) plus one nonnucleoside reverse transcriptase inhibitor (NNRTI), while 22 percent of patients received two NRTIs plus a protease inhibitor. ART in this program was provided on a patient copayment basis. For example, the MOPH supplied either efavirenz or ritonavir-boosted indinavir for free, and the patient purchased the two backbone nucleoside drugs to make up a triple antiretroviral combination.

In parallel to the development of the ATC program, the government decided to strengthen national capacity to manufacture a variety of off-patent antiretroviral drugs. Generic production of antiretroviral drugs by the Government Pharmaceutical Organization (GPO) significantly reduced their price in Thailand (table 2.2). Most important, GPO started to produce a single-tablet triple-drug combination regimen called GPO-vir (stavudine + lamivudine + nevirapine) at a price of US$30 (B 1,200) per month.[7] With the availability of the GPO-vir single-tablet combination regimen in 2002, the ATC program was upgraded, and GPO-vir became the first-line regimen for treating naive patients. The availability of a low-priced generic ART in a

**Table 2.2**  Declining Minimum Prices of ART in Thailand

| ART triple-drug regimen | Year | Price (B per month)[a] |
|---|---|---|
| 2 NRTIs + PI | Before 2000 | > 25,000 |
| 2 NRTIs + boosted PI | 2000 | 13,000 |
|  | 2002 | 6,000 |
| 2 NRTIs + NNRTI | Before 2000 | 15,000 |
|  | Early 2001 | 13,000 |
|  | Mid-2001 | < 6,000 |
|  | Late 2001 | 2,300 |
| GPO-vir | 2002 | 1,200 |
| GPO-vir | 2004 | 1,200 |

Source: Phoolcharoen and others 2004b.
Note: NRTI = nucleoside reverse transcriptase inhibitor; NNRTI = nonnucleoside reverse transcriptase inhibitor; PI = protease inhibitor.
a. These are the minimum prices for drugs in Thailand in the public sector. Actual prices paid may vary significantly.

triple-drug combination suddenly opened the possibility of large-scale provision of ART to eligible patients (table 2.2).

The pilot ATC initiative was first evaluated in several hospitals in six northern provinces in 2001 (Leusaree and others 2002). From February to October 2001, 774 adult HIV patients in 54 district and provincial hospitals enrolled into the program. The mean CD4 count at commencement of ART was 84 cells cells per cubic millimeter. After 24 weeks, 68.6 percent were still on treatment. Reasons for stopping therapy were

- adverse events (101 patients, or 13.1 percent of the cohort)

- death (41 patients, or 5.3 percent)

- nonspecified treatment failure (42 patients, or 5.4 percent)

- loss to follow-up (35 patients, or 4.5 percent)

- other (24 patients, or 3.1 percent).

A parallel rapid assessment of the ATC program in northern Thailand found even greater dropout rates (of about 45 percent) (Community Medicine Department, Chiang Mai University 2002). Both evaluations concluded that significant improvements in the program were needed to ensure greater adherence. Areas identified for improvement included

- the need for ongoing capacity building in ART management among health care providers, especially nurses and pharmacists

- a strengthened role for counselors

- greater involvement of family and community in ART delivery and support for patients.

*Scale-up of National Access to ART Program*
In 2003, the Thai government expanded the ATC program with a four-year commitment (2003–6) to provide triple-drug ART as a standard of care. The objective of this program, named the National Access to Antiretrovirals Program for People Living with HIV/AIDS, or NAPHA, was to provide access by the end of 2004 to triple-drug ART to a large proportion of all persons living with symptomatic HIV/AIDS. The number of PHAs on ART increased from about 3,000 at the start of 2002 to 27,000 by the end of 2003 and to 52,000 by February 2005. The program is financed in part with funds from the Global Fund to Fight AIDS, Tuberculosis, and Malaria (GFATM) and in part with government budget funds. The number of treatment sites increased from 112 in 2001 to 462 in early 2003 and to 841 by February 2005.

Table 2.3 shows the evolution of estimated cases of PHAs, AIDS cases, and access to public ART in Thailand. As of the end of 2004, more than 80 percent of those living with AIDS had access to public ART—a remarkable achievement. Figure 2.8 plots those trends, illustrating that

**Table 2.3** Estimated Cases of People Living with AIDS, AIDS Cases, Reported AIDS Cases in Public Hospitals, and Access to Public ART

| Type of case | 1997 | 1998 | 1999 | 2000 | 2001 | 2002 | 2003 | 2004 |
|---|---|---|---|---|---|---|---|---|
| People living with HIV/AIDS | 751,235 | 740,349 | 719,765 | 649,564 | 665,344 | 635,057 | 603,942 | 572,484 |
| People living with AIDS | 59,752 | 65,333 | 68,311 | 68,677 | 67,057 | 64,832 | 62,871 | 61,394 |
| People using ART from public care | 1,095[a] | 1,095[a] | 1,095[a] | 2,095[a] | 2,095[a] | 8,341[a] | 27,158 | 52,593[b] |
| Percentage of AIDS cases in public ART | 1.8 | 1.7 | 1.6 | 3.1 | 3.1 | 12.9 | 43.2 | 81.4 |
| Percentage of reported AIDS in public ART | 4.1 | 4.0 | 4.0 | 4.5 | 8.5 | 35.5 | 122.6 | — |

*Source:* Thai Working Group on HIV/AIDS Projection 2001; Gold and others 2004; MOPH 2004.
*Note:* — = not available.
a. Follow-up to the *Declaration of Commitment of HIV/AIDS (UNGASS) Country Report* 2002.
b. Figures are as of February 2005. The data were provided by the Bureau of AIDS. TB, and STI at MOPH (2004)

**Figure 2.8**  People Living with AIDS and Public ART Provision

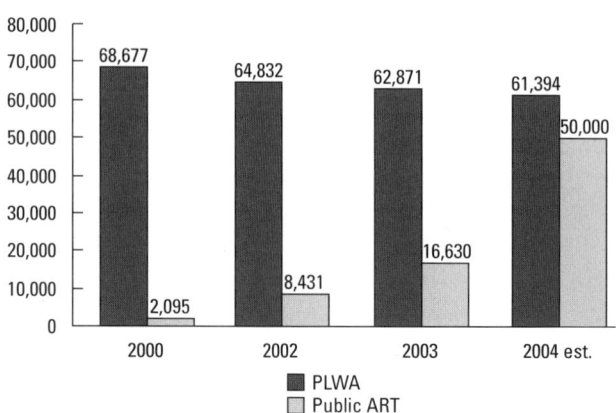

*Source:* Thai Working Group on HIV/AIDS Projection 2001; Gold and others 2005. Clinical Background Paper for Expanding Access to ART in Thailand Report 2004; MOPH 2004. The data were provided to the authors by the Bureau of AIDS. TB, and STI at MOPH 2004.

the proportion of people living with AIDS in Thailand with access to public ART has increased sixfold since 2002.

Table 2.4 shows the number of people on public ART by region as of March 2004, as well as the ART targets that MOPH set for the end of 2004. These targets were calculated as a function of the estimated number of AIDS and symptomatic HIV cases in the corresponding region (as reported by the hospital system for reporting AIDS cases). The table shows that some regions have come closer to reaching their targets than others: the north and the northeast have the highest ratios of people on ART relative to their targets. This finding may

**Table 2.4**  Number of Patients on ART in Thailand by Region, March 2004

| Region | Accumulated patients[a] | Current patients on ART | New patients | Target in 2004 |
|---|---|---|---|---|
| Bangkok | 2,846 | 2,648 | 272 | 5,830 |
| Central | 7,491 | 6,749 | 1,537 | 16,240 |
| North | 8,777 | 7,459 | 1,030 | 11,648 |
| Northeast | 7,643 | 6,983 | 1,461 | 8,673 |
| South | 3,232 | 2,825 | 213 | 6,109 |
| Other (PHPT) | 494 | 494 | — | 1,500 |
| Total | 30,483 | 27,158 | 4,513 | 50,000 |

*Source:* MOPH 2004.
*Note:* PHPT = Program for HIV Prevention and Treatment (PHPT): Clinical trials on the prevention of mother to child transmission of HIV; — = not available.
a. Accumulated from ATC 2000 up to NAPHA, March 2004.

reflect the fact that those regions saw an earlier expansion of ART and have larger numbers of facilities providing ART, or it could reflect higher uptake rates. The figures do not allow us to distinguish between those possibilities.

Map 2.3, located in the Maps section at the end of the book, presents a spatial illustration of the expansion of ART in Thailand by showing the distribution of current ART patients and that of symptomatic HIV patients (a proxy for the implicit target population for ART) by province, as of March 2004. Map 2.4 gives a slightly different perspective on coverage by showing the distribution of symptomatic HIV patients against province-level ART coverage (district-level data on ART are not available).

Anecdotal evidence, as well as conversations with the MOPH, suggests that contrary to what may be expected, little rationing of access to public ART has taken place. Many hospitals in parts of the country report not using all the ART treatment slots allocated to them. This lack of rationing could exist because hospital capacity to deliver ART is stretched in other ways (for example, scarce human resources able and willing to deliver ART); it may be that people living with AIDS are not going to the public health facilities for care or are going only once they are very sick. Stigma, discrimination, and a desire not to self-disclose could work against PHAs coming in for treatment. Access to publicly provided ART requires PHAs to disclose their status to their local district hospital. Fear of discrimination for themselves and their families could prompt many to seek treatment outside their districts, from other district hospitals, or from the private sector (see, for example, the case presented in chapter 1, box 1.1). In both cases, PHAs would have to pay for ART out of pocket, which could impose a sizable financial burden.

Interviews with PHAs in different regions suggest that discrimination and stigma may be a factor, but many PHAs pointed also to the lack of readiness of providers in some hospitals to be involved in ART as a major barrier to access. Financial barriers are also mentioned as an important factor, particularly for those who are not part of the "30-Baht" scheme (the UCS, or Universal Coverage Scheme) (Phongphit 2004). Even for those who are covered under the UCS and entitled to free ART drugs, costs may be sizable; typically, monitoring tests (in particular, CD4 counts and viral-load tests) are not free and can be quite costly. The price of CD4 testing by standard flow cytometry varies from B 200 to B 800 (US\$5 to US\$20), depending on the institution providing it (see chapter 3). The price of a viral load test can be as high as B 3,500 (US$90). A basic safety chemistry panel—testing SGOT (serum glutamic oxaloacetic transaminase), creatinine, and glucose—costs B 100 (US$2.50). Lack of information about ART is cited as another significant barrier to access (Phongpit 2004).

Enrollment in the national ART program has been voluntary for hospitals, and many have elected not to join or elected to take only a very small quota of patients. Map 2.5 gives yet another perspective on the expansion of NAPHA by showing the increase in the number of health facilities providing ART. The total number went from 112 in 2001 to 462 in 2002; it increased further to 841 facilities by the end of 2003. The expansion of facilities providing ART between 2001 and 2003 correlates geographically with the distribution of cumulative AIDS and symptomatic HIV cases. Map 2.6 shows the average number of ART participants per enrolled NAPHA hospital. The hospitals handling the largest numbers of patients per facility are located in Bangkok and in the north.

*Augmented Public ART*

In addition to those accessing ART through the public system, a limited number of PHAs are receiving treatment at public hospitals in an "augmented" setting, with the active support of nongovernment institutions such as Médecins sans Frontières (MSF) and the Thai Red Cross and the HIV–Netherlands Australia Thailand Research Collaboration (HIV-NAT) and greater involvement of PHA peer support groups. MSF, for example, has been working with three district hospitals in Thailand since 2000 to provide care for about 330 patients on ART. Estimates suggest that about 1,800 patients are receiving this augmented ART (table 2.5).

In the MSF model, patient care is the responsibility of the district hospital and is provided by a nurse-managed multidisciplinary team. The team includes doctors, pharmacists, nurses, lab technicians, and PHA peer counselors. The team leader is usually a senior nurse with sufficient experience and authority to manage staff members from other disciplines. Because doctors in district hospitals are extremely busy— one doctor is often responsible for as many as 100 outpatient consultations daily as well as wards and the emergency room—not all patients taking ART see the doctor at every appointment. Patients are referred to doctors for adverse reactions or suspicion of opportunistic infection. In this setting, the PHA peer counselors have many important roles:

- informing their community about availability of treatment

- giving basic information to clients in easy-to-understand language

- discussing treatment plans and disclosure

- solving problems in case of practical difficulties with adherence

- visiting clients at home in case of loss to follow-up.

In addition to supplying drugs, MSF provides ongoing support that includes shared consultations and home visits, case conferences, and training for both hospital staff members and PHAs (Wilson and Ford 2004).

Patients receiving ART in this augmented public setting are likely to benefit from more active counseling and support from other PHAs than those receiving ART without the benefit of NGO involvement. The expectation is that this augmentation will help sustain adherence. Indeed, experience over the past three years at MSF indicates that PHAs can make a large contribution in supporting adherence to treatment. This contribution comes from the willingness of PHA to help their peers and share their experiences, but the necessary training and coordination demands long-term funding and ongoing technical support. Given the low level of education of PHAs in general, particular attention needs to be given to developing an easy-to-use, reliable reporting system (Wilson and Ford 2004).

Since October 2003, TNP+ (the Thai Network of People Living with AIDS), MSF, and the AIDS Access Foundation have been cooperating to prepare PHA groups further for a role to support the government's rapid scale-up of ART. In May 2004, the beneficiaries of this project were 104 PHA groups working alongside hospital staff, according to

**Table 2.5** Number of Patients on ART by Type of Provider, March 2004

| Type of provider | Accumulated patients | Current patients on ART | MOPH target |
|---|---|---|---|
| Public | 47,100 | 40,939 | 50,000 |
| Augmented public | 2,000 | 1,800 | |
| Private | — | — | — |
| Total on ART | 49,100 | 42,739 | 50,000 |
| Not on ART | 12,294 | 18,650 | |
| People living with AIDS | 61,394 | 61,394 | 61,394 |

Source: Data for public providers are from the MOPH; data for augmented public providers are estimated on the basis of numbers provide by MSF, HIV-NAT, and the MOPH; data for private providers are not available.

the model described above, in the three MSF pilot hospitals. The geographic distribution of these PHA groups is shown in map 2.7. Most of the funding for this effort is provided by the GFATM as part of Thailand's successful first-round application. The MOPH's goal is that eventually all public hospitals providing ART will actively engage PHA peer counselors and support groups. However, for this PHA role to be sustainable, long-term funding and ongoing technical support will be essential, and the government will need to facilitate liaison between PHA representatives and hospitals.

The work of PHAs has been a valuable contribution to the government's rapid scale-up of ART. The change in PHAs' involvement in health care from receiver to coprovider has led to improved acceptance of and support for PHAs within the health care system. Increased control over their health has also brought benefits for PHAs in terms of self-image, confidence, and dignity. MSF acts as a bridge between PHAs, donors, and the government. This work, which has addressed both practical and political obstacles, has succeeded in part because PHAs maintained the space to develop their own priorities. The partnership with other national groups and international organizations has been successful because of an understanding among all involved that the relationship is one of equals.

*Private Access to ART*

Data on private access to ART in Thailand are relatively scarce, with no direct data from private providers available. However, because the GPO sells a share of its GPO-vir triple-drug combination tablet directly to the private sector through several retail centers in Bangkok, figures on those sales can be used as a proxy for private sector access. This information is synthesized in table 2.6, which shows the share of sales of GPO-vir to the public, domestic private, and pri-

**Table 2.6**  Sales of GPO-vir by Sector, 2002–4

| Sector | 2002 | 2003 | 2004 (projected) | Total (projected) |
|--------|------|------|------------------|-------------------|
| Public | 58.2 | 78.2 | 82.2 | 80.5 |
| Private domestic | 39.9 | 20.0 | 15.9 | 17.7 |
| Private international | 1.9 | 1.8 | 1.9 | 1.8 |
| Total | 100.0 | 100.0 | 100.0 | 100.0 |
| For memo: | | | | |
| Total volume of sales | 44,415 | 283,894 | 929,656 | 1,257,965 |

*Source:* Data from Thailand's Government Pharmaceutical Office provided by the MOPH to the authors in 2004.

vate international sectors for 2002 to 2004. According to these figures, roughly 20 percent of total sales of GPO-vir in 2003 went to the private domestic sector (down from about 40 percent in 2002). This share was projected to decline further, to about 16 percent, by the end of 2004. Private international sales for 2004 were expected to remain constant at about 2 percent of the total.

According to MOPH officials, ART cannot be dispensed outside a hospital setting by private doctors. However, private hospitals in Bangkok and other major cities can and do provide ART, typically on an out-of-pocket payment basis. Many doctors working in public or university settings report seeing patients privately, but no representative nationwide figures can be used to estimate the scale of private sector delivery. The only evidence comes from a survey of Thai physicians that was conducted in January 2004 at a Thai Red Cross and HIV-NAT conference on HIV/AIDS management for practicing clinicians and health care staff. This survey was given to some 84 practicing AIDS clinicians from a wide range of clinical and geographic settings (see Gold and others 2004).

Survey results from these doctors, many of whom practiced in both the private and the public sectors, suggest that only about 18 percent of patients were seen privately. The survey revealed few differences in patient characteristics at the start of ART whether the physician practiced in the private, public, or academic sector. Most patients were generally very immunosuppressed (66 percent with CD4 counts of less than 100 cells per microliter) and symptomatic (68 percent). About 60 percent were on ART, with most taking GPO-vir or other first-line therapies. Very few patients were taking protease inhibitor–based regimens (13 percent), and about 30 percent were not on ART but receiving treatment or prophylaxis for opportunistic infections.[8]

## AIDS Expenditure and Financing

Thai health policy makers have been working to expand insurance coverage to the Thai population while ensuring the financial soundness of the government health care system. In this context, the government's decision to finance AIDS care raises issues regarding the sustainability of the overall health care financing system and whether AIDS care should be financed in the same way as care for other health problems.

## *Health Care Coverage for AIDS Prevention and Treatment*

The four main health insurance schemes cover nearly 100 percent of the population:

- The Social Security Scheme (SSS) and Workmen's Compensation Fund (WCF) cover formal private sector workers.

- The Civil Servant Medical Benefit Scheme (CSMBS) covers government employees.

- The "30-baht" or Universal Coverage Scheme covers the rest of the population.

The characteristics and scope of each program are described in table 2.7. The schemes are managed independently, with different reimbursement mechanisms and separate reporting requirements for providers.

The largest scheme is the UCS, which was introduced on a national scale in April 2002 with the aim of guaranteeing access to health care to every Thai citizen, regardless of income and means. The UCS replaced all previous schemes targeted to the poor and uninsured. Evidence from its operation during 2002 to 2004 suggests that it has succeeded in

- increasing health care coverage from about 70 percent of the population before its introduction to nearly 100 percent

- significantly increasing health care use, particularly of outpatient services, while reducing out-of-pocket expenditures by households.

These increases and decreases have been proportionally largest for those in the bottom two quintiles of the income distribution, suggesting that the UCS is significantly pro-poor.

Despite these accomplishments, broad agreement exists on two points:

- Existing capitation rates under the UCS are too low.

- The system is underfunded.

The impact of this underfunding is partly dampened by cross-subsidization at the provider level from the other health insurance

**Table 2.7** Health Insurance Schemes in Thailand

| Characteristics | SSS and WCF | CSMBS | UCS ("30-baht") |
|---|---|---|---|
| Model | Public contracted | Public reimbursement | Public contracted |
| Population covered | Private formal sector employees, but not their dependents (establishments with more than 10 workers): 8 million | Government employees and their dependents: 4.5 million | People not covered by SSS or CSMBS: 47 million |
| **Benefit package** | | | |
| Ambulatory services | Public and private | Public only | Registered public and private |
| Inpatient services | Public and private | Public and private | Registered public and private |
| Choice of provider | Contracted hospital or its network, registration required | Free choice | Registration required |
| Types of benefits | Non-work-related illnesses, injuries (work-related covered under WCF) | Comprehensive package | Comprehensive package |
| **Financing** | | | |
| Source of funds | Contributions from employees, employers, and government amounting to 4.5 percent of insurable earnings payroll | General tax revenues | General tax revenues |
| Financing body | Social Security Office (SSO) | Ministry of Finance | National Health Security Office (NHSO) |
| Payment mechanism | Capitation | Fee for service | 2 options: inclusive capitation for inpatient, outpatient, and preventive and health promotion; (ii) or capitation for outpatient and preventive and health promotion; Diagnosis Related Group (DRG) with global budget for inpatient |
| Copayment | Maternity, emergency services if above ceiling | Yes, if inpatient at private hospital | Yes, 30 baht per visit. No copay for inpatient. |
| Expenditures per capita | B 1,558 (in 1999) | B 2,106 (in 1999) | B 1,202 (in 2003) |

*Source:* Jogudomsuk and others 2003.

schemes (especially CSMBS). However, over time—and especially as cost containment efforts in CSMBS take effect—the financial squeeze on UCS providers is expected to tighten, which could lead to deteriorating quality. Current programming and budgeting practices for the UCS—with capitation rates set annually on the basis of available budget resources—make its funding highly vulnerable to cyclical downturns and swings in tax revenues. Over the long term, such practices may undermine its financial sustainability.

In addition to financial constraints, scarcity of human resources, especially physicians, may present a problem for the sustainability of the UCS system in its present form. Increased health care use in a limited-resource context has sharply increased workloads for the staff in the public health system. Indeed, since the introduction of the UCS in 2002, the number of physicians leaving the public system because of increased workloads and low pay has accelerated. The rapid scale-up of ART will add substantially to these pressures.

The different schemes offer slightly different coverage and quality of care for PHAs. The UCS covers preventive and curative care (treatment of all opportunistic infections) but does not cover ART or associated testing and monitoring. Access to ART for PHAs covered by the UCS is offered under NAPHA, which is run as a separate vertical program under the MOPH. ART is available for all PHAs who meet the eligibility criteria and present for treatment at their registered hospitals (assuming the hospital has a treatment slot available; some regions have waiting lists). The patient must pay for the first CD4 test (about B 500), but all monitoring and testing after enrollment is covered by NAPHA, as is the cost of the drugs. In practice, however, hospitals exercise some discretion in asking patients to copay, depending on an assessment of their means.

Discussion continues among policy makers and politicians about the desirability of integrating ART treatment into the UCS. The political commitment to include ART in the package has been made explicit on several occasions by the minister of public health—and recently, at the July 2004 Bangkok International AIDS conference, by the prime minister himself. Indeed, it is expected that ART will be included under the UCS soon.

Until August 2004, NAPHA also covered access to ART for PHA under the SSS. As under the UCS, SSS patients were required to pay for the first CD4 count, but all subsequent monitoring and testing, as well as the cost of the ART, was covered by NAPHA (although, again, with discretion on the part of the hospitals for copayments). All other inpatient and outpatient care for PHA was covered by SSS. As of August 2004, the SSS includes access to ART as part of its care package for PHAs. All SSS patients being treated under NAPHA will thus be transferred to SSS (about 13,000). Guidelines for treatment (including the choice of drug regimens for first-line treatment) are purported to be similar for SSS and NAPHA. The CSMBS covers all PHA care including ART and associated monitoring and testing.

## Trends in AIDS Expenditure

According to the National AIDS Accounts (Teokul and others 2005), total health expenditure on HIV/AIDS increased from B 2.996 billion in 2000 (US$74.4 million) to B 4.188 billion in 2003 (US$101.3 million). The largest increases in spending during this period came from the ART program (which more than tripled in spending) and from outpatient care (table 2.8). In response, the share of total AIDS

**Table 2.8** National AIDS Expenditure by Function, 2000–2003

| Functions | 2000 | 2001 | 2002 | 2003 |
|---|---|---|---|---|
| Current health spending (B million) | 2,690 | 2,922 | 3,154 | 3,999.6 |
| Inpatient care | 687.1 | 715.7 | 432.5 | 431.6 |
| Outpatient care | 836.5 | 928.4 | 1,010 | 1,033 |
| ART | 606.9 | 797.1 | 1,242.9 | 2.099 |
| PMTCT | 210.8 | 188.7 | 184.2 | 140.1 |
| VCT | 28.5 | 27.6 | 24.9 | 39.5 |
| Blood safety | 84.3 | 84.3 | 84.3 | 84.3 |
| Condom program | 49.4 | 35.5 | 69.7 | 42.2 |
| AIDS education | 21.7 | 36.2 | 29.5 | 41.3 |
| IDU harm reduction | 100.2 | 28.1 | 59.3 | 73.4 |
| Surveillance | 19.1 | 18.0 | 16.9 | 15.2 |
| Program administration | 45.5 | 63.2 | — | — |
| Health care–related expenditure (research and development, training) | 201.1 | 104.9 | 5.49 | 102.7 |
| Total (B million) | 2,996.0 | 3,312.4 | 3,253.5 | 4,188.0 |
| Total (US$ million) | 74.4 | 70.4 | 75.9 | 101.3 |

*Source:* Teokul and others 2005.
*Note:* — = not available.

expenditure going to ART increased from 20.3 percent in 2000 to 50.1 percent in 2003. Jointly, ART and treatment of opportunistic infections account for 85.1 percent of total AIDS spending. The share of spending going to prevention activities has declined sharply, from 9.3 percent in 2000 to 5.1 percent in 2003, but the level has remained roughly constant in current prices. Within the prevention budget, the sharpest decline in both share and levels has occurred in harm reduction activities for IDUs.

## Sources of Financing

Most expenditures on HIV/AIDS have been financed from public budgetary sources, which accounted for about 65 to 80 percent of total AIDS expenditure during 2000 to 2003 (figure 2.9). The share of financing coming from the two main health insurance schemes, SSS and CSMBS, has remained stable at about 2.5 percent and 3 percent, respectively, for the same period. However, the share of spending by SSS is expected to increase; the scheme recently started to cover ART. Under this new policy, about 13,000 patients are expected to shift from NAPHA to SSS. Household out-of-pocket spending has also played a significant role in financing AIDS expenditures, accounting for 27 to 28 percent of total AIDS spending. Other donor sources played a negligible role until 2003, when resources from the GFATM started to kick in, raising the share of financing by external sources to about 9 percent of the total.[9]

**Figure 2.9** Sources of HIV/AIDS Program Financing, 2000–2003

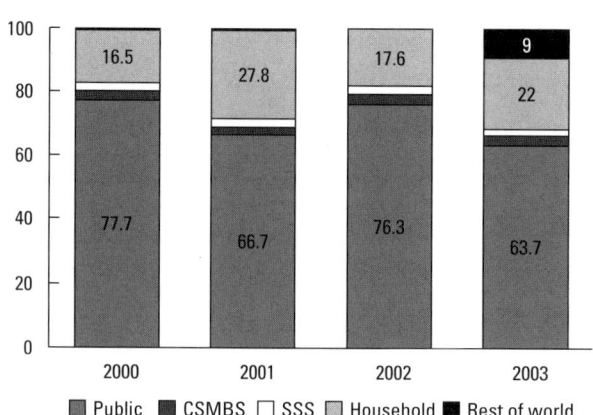

Source: Teokul and others 2005.

**Figure 2.10**  National AIDS Budget Allocation, 1996–2004

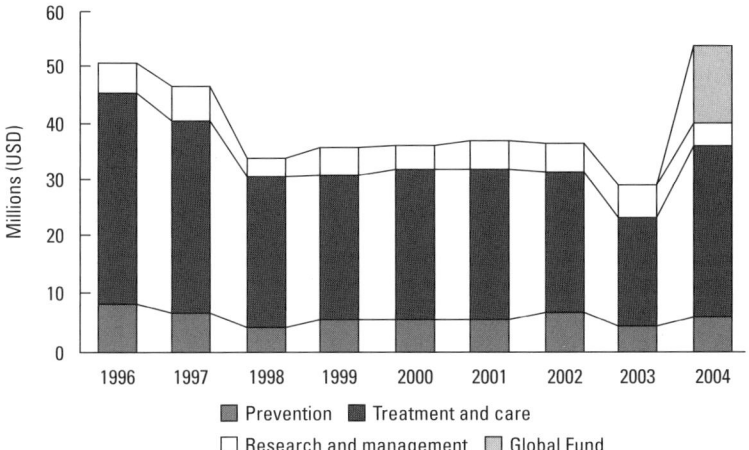

Source: MOPH, National Prevention and Alleviation of AIDS Budget Allocation by the Royal Thai Government 2004; Bureau of AIDS, TB, and STI at MOPH 2004; MOPH 2004.

## National Budget Allocations for AIDS Prevention and Treatment

Figure 2.10 shows the evolution of the national AIDS budget for the period 1996–2003. The patterns in the budget allocation parallel those reflected in the National AIDS Accounts—namely an increase in the level and share of expenditures on treatment and care, of which the largest share is due to ART, and a slight reduction in the share and level of prevention spending.

### Notes

1.   HIV prevalence refers to the stock of existing infections at a point in time; HIV incidence refers to the flow of new HIV infections at a given period of time. Greater access to ART has changed the dynamics of the AIDS epidemic. HIV prevalence can decline either with more deaths among AIDS patients or with fewer new infections among the population. Successful scale-up of ART would increase HIV prevalence as a result of both delays in AIDS deaths and increased life expectancy with treatment. In the era of universal access to ART, incidence rate is a better measure of prevention success than prevalence rate.

2. On average in Thailand, the delay between infection with HIV and the onset of AIDS is 7 to 10 years (see chapter 3).

3. This scarcity is unfortunate because these socioeconomic determinants of HIV infection are also likely to affect demand for voluntary counseling and testing and ART, as well as have an influence on adherence.

4. This section draws heavily from an earlier World Bank study (World Bank 2000); from a background paper on policy development prepared by the Bureau of AIDS, Tuberculosis, and STIs, the Department of Disease Control of the Ministry of Health (Thanprasertsuk and others 2004); and from the UNDP thematic Millennium Devlopment Goal report on AIDS (Phoolcharoen and others 2004a).

5. The HIV surveillance survey was originally carried out twice a year, but since the decline in new infections in 1995, it has been conducted only once a year (in June) among five major target groups. At the time of writing, the most recent survey had taken place in June 2003.

6. This section draws on Duncombe (2004) and Thanprasertsuk (2004).

7. The price of GPO-vir has not changed since 2002, unlike the prices of other generic triple-drug combinations produced by manufacturers in India.

8. A second round of the Thai physicians' survey was carried out in January 2005 at the annual Thai Red Cross and HIV-NAT conference. The data have been processed but still need to be analyzed.

9. Although the World Bank has been a major funder of AIDS prevention interventions, Thailand has never sought World Bank financial support for AIDS prevention or treatment.

# CHAPTER 3

# HIV/AIDS and Antiretroviral Therapy

This chapter presents some of the basic principles of HIV biology as a foundation for a discussion of the cost-effectiveness of treatment alternatives and of their intended and unintended consequences.

## Natural History of HIV Infection without Antiretroviral Therapy

Epidemiologists use the term *natural history* to describe the sequence of symptoms and biological events that occur in the average untreated person suffering from a disease, from onset to recovery or death.

### Biological Markers of HIV Disease

The natural history of HIV disease is one of a relentless battle between HIV and the immune system that results in progressive destruction of the body's capacity to fight serious infections and cancers. The period between infection and illness can be as short as a few weeks to as long as a few months, but in most cases, illness begins to seriously affect quality of life and economic potential within a median time of seven years. Once the characteristic opportunistic infections (OIs) or cancers emerge, which determine when the patient is classified as having AIDS, life expectancy declines sharply. Elements that influence the pace of disease progression include virulence of HIV; genetic, nutritional, and general health factors of the host; and access to therapies that ameliorate viral production (antiretroviral therapy) and mitigate the effects of OIs.

The most indicative biological marker of HIV disease progression is a decline in the number of CD4 cells (also known as *T4-helper cells*) in the blood. CD4 cells are critical to the body's immune response. When HIV enters the body, it binds itself to the CD4 cells, combines with the DNA in the cell nucleus, and eventually destroys the cells. At the initial infection stage, the level of circulating virus (viral load) is very high, and the CD4 count temporarily drops. However, soon after the initial infection stage, a balance is usually reached between the degree of viral replication and the immune control system that allows the CD4 count to recuperate. Over time, though, HIV progressively destroys the immune system until the CD4 count may drop to zero. As the CD4 cells become depleted, their function of protecting the body from a range of viral, fungal, and mycobacterial agents and tumors also declines to such low levels that those diseases cannot be controlled. At that stage, the body becomes highly susceptible to OIs and cancers (Gold and others 2005). An established relationship exists between the level of CD4 cells in the blood and the risk of development of OIs. In general, a CD4 count of less than 200 cells per cubic millimeter is regarded as the threshold for high risk for developing serious illnesses. As the CD4 count declines further, an increasing number of OIs begins to manifest, the most serious starting to appear when the CD4 count drops below 50 cells per cubic millimeter. A person's CD4 count is the best predictive marker of mortality associated with HIV disease. That count is also the best indicator of response to antiretroviral therapy (ART).

### The Natural History of HIV in Thailand

Few fundamental differences can be identified between the natural history of HIV in Thailand and the history observed in most other middle-level or developed countries. In a large, prospective cohort study of HIV progression in Thailand, follow-up data on 757 HIV-infected patients indicated that progression rates are similar to those observed in cohorts in Australia, Europe, and the United States (Wannamethee and others 1998). However, other studies suggest that progression rates in Thailand may be more rapid than in Western cohorts. Table 3.1 presents a summary of those results. The data confirm that CD4 count is the most important single indicator of disease progression. For example, the table shows that 47.1 percent of the 169 HIV-infected patients with a first CD4 count of less than 200 cells per cubic millimeter developed AIDS within one year, as compared with 6.6 percent of those with an initial CD4 count of between 200 and 499 cells per cubic millimeter and as compared with 6.0 percent of those with a CD4 count above 500 cells per cubic millimeter. The table also shows that men progressed to AIDS somewhat faster that women and that increasing age was associated with HIV disease progression and mortality.

In a second natural history cohort study, 235 young Thai army recruits, whose seroconversion date was known, were followed for at least five years to determine progression to AIDS and death. Only two men in that cohort ever received ART, and in both cases, it was zidovudine (AZT) monotherapy. Also, only two men received treatment for latent tuberculosis (TB), and 12 men received trimethoprim-sulfamethoxazole prophylaxis for pneumocystis carinii pneumonia (PCP). Hence, that study may be as close to a natural history cohort as exists in Thailand. The mortality rate was found to be 56.3 deaths per 1,000 person years, nine times that of the HIV-negative controls. The five-year mortality rate of around 18 percent was twice as high as that of Western country cohorts. The median time to AIDS for those men, who were generally in the 15- to 24-year-old group, was 7.4 years, which is substantially less than that found in the analysis of natural history studies in Western countries.[1] The investigators also calculated the time from seroconversion to the first CD4 count of less than 200 cells per cubic millimeter, in order to estimate the time for optimal commencement of ART. That calculation revealed a period of 6.9 years, which was comparable to the time-to-AIDS calculation. The authors (Chin and others 2001) also calculated the 7-year AIDS-free rate of 57.0 percent, which indicates that HIV disease progressed relatively rapidly in that cohort compared with cohorts in Western countries.

In an attempt to explain those observations, the investigators (Chin and others 2001) note that the HIV viral load in their cohort at seroconversion was much higher than that found in other cohorts from Western countries. They also noted that the high viral load persisted for the first six months before settling to a level comparable to the Western cohorts after 12 months. They hypothesized that this very high viral load may influence the rate of disease progression and may, in some way, be related to infection with HIV subtype E, which is found in more than 95 percent of sexually transmitted HIV in Thailand. In another interesting observation to explain rapid progression rates, the investigators note the baseline CD4 count at seroconversion was a mean of 764

**Table 3.1** Selected Characteristics and Disease Progression Rates in a Cohort of HIV-Infected Patients Managed at Chulalongkorn University Hospital, Thailand, 1998

| Characteristic | Number of patients | Median CD4 count (cells/mm³) | Rate per 100 person years observed (%) | Relative risk (confidence interval) unadjusted/adjusted for initial CD4 count |
|---|---|---|---|---|
| All | 757 | 324 | 12.2 | |
| *CD4 count (cells/mm³)* | | | | |
| < 200 | 169 | 93 | 47.1 | 9.1 (5.4–16.0) |
| 200–499 | 366 | 343 | 6.6 | 1.3 (0.7–2.3) |
| 500+ | 222 | 713 | 6.0 | 1.0 |
| *Risk group* | | | | |
| Heterosexual | 562 | 321 | 11.7 | 1.0 |
| Homosexual | 104 | 501 | 13.6 | 1.1 (0.7–1.9)/2.4 (1.4–4.0) |
| Injecting drug users | 57 | 480 | 13.4 | 1.1 (0.5–2.4)/1.8 (0.9–3.9) |
| Other | 19 | 588 | 6.9 | 0.6 (0.1–2.5)/1.8 (0.4–7.5) |
| *Sex* | | | | |
| Male | 644 | 355 | 13.1 | 1.0 |
| Female | 113 | 384 | 5.4 | 0.4 (0.2–0.9)/0.4 (0.2–1.0) |
| *Age at entry* | | | | |
| < 20 | 23 | 471 | 0 | 1.0 |
| 20–29 | 343 | 373 | 10.8 | 1.4 (0.9–2.2)/1.1 (0.7–1.8) |
| 30–39 | 233 | 324 | 13.7 | 1.6 (0.9–2.7)/1.3 (0.7–2.3) |
| 40–49 | 115 | 332 | 14.5 | |
| Antiretrovirals (usually zidovudine) | | | | |
| No | 452 | 456 | 9.2 | 1.0 |
| Yes | 305 | 277 | 15.5 | 1.7(1.2–2.5)/0.9(0.7–1.7) |

*Source:* Adapted from Wannamethee and others 1998.

cells per cubic millimeter compared with a mean of 988 cells per cubic millimeter seen in the Multicenter AIDS Cohort Study in the United States (Enger and others 1996). That lower initial CD4 count in the Thai cohort may account for the early drop of CD4 to less than 200 cells per cubic millimeter, because the baseline is lower.

One of the most relevant markers of disease progression is the rate of CD4 cell destruction. A recent retrospective cohort study, which was conducted as part of the background research for this study at Siriraj University Hospital, suggests that the decline in CD4 counts among infected persons from Thailand mirrors observations in industrial countries of about 50 to 70 cells per year (Ratanasuwan 2004). That situation is illustrated in figure 3.1.

**Figure 3.1**   Decline in CD4 Count by Year of Follow-Up, Siriraj University Hospital, Thailand

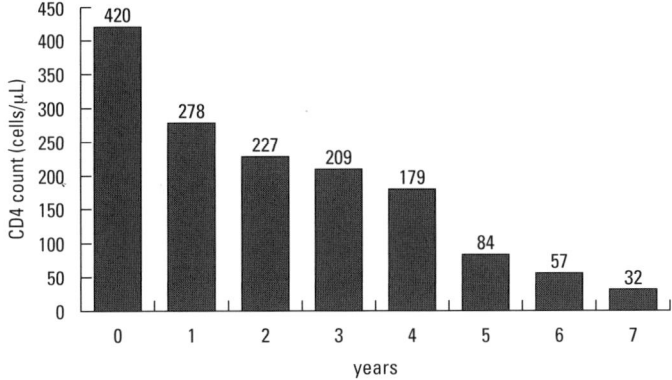

*Source:* Ratanasuwan 2004.
*Note: n* = 117; mean follow-up is 48 months.

## *Transmission of HIV in Various Risk Groups*

The main modes of transmission of HIV are well described and are documented both in a broad context and for Thailand in particular (MOPH and Division of Epidemiology various years; Phoolcharoen and others 2004b; World Bank 2000). A range of transmission risks by mode of transmission, drawn from worldwide experience (Royce and others 1997), is presented in table 3.2.

**Table 3.2**   Average Transmission Risk of HIV by Mode of Transmission

| Mode of transmission | Risk of infection |
|---|---|
| *Sexual intercourse* | |
| Female-to-male transmission | 1 in 700 to 1 in 3,000 |
| Male-to-female transmission | 1 in 200 to 1 in 2,000 |
| Male-to-male transmission | 1 in 10 to 1 in 1,600 |
| Fellatio | 1 in 13 to 1 in 17 |
| *Needles* | |
| Needle stick | 1 in 200 |
| Needle sharing | 1 in 150 |
| Transfusion of infected blood | 95 in 100 |
| *Transmission from mother to infant* | |
| Without AZT treatment | 1 in 3–5 |
| With AZT treatment | < 1 in 10 |
| Combination ART | 1 in 50 |

*Source:* Adapted from Royce and others 1997.

Those are the average risks. However, for any particular individual, the specific risk of contracting HIV may vary significantly, depending on the combination of factors present at the time of exposure. The most critical aspects are the infectiousness of the infected person, which is positively correlated with his or her viral load, and the susceptibility of the person exposed, which is higher if the person has an ulcerative sexually transmitted infection (STI), is the receptive partner in sexual intercourse, or is an uncircumcised male. Different types of HIV may also have different capacities for infection. Subtype C, not prevalent in Thailand, is thought to be the most infectious.

## Treatment of Opportunistic Infections with or without ART

Even as the availability of ART increases in many developing countries, appropriate diagnosis and management of life-threatening OIs and HIV-associated cancers still remain the most important aspects of the care of patients with HIV disease. OIs and cancers usually begin at least five to seven years after infection and occur progressively as uncontrolled HIV replication destroys the immune system (Colebunders and Latif 1991; Muñoz, Sabin, and Phillips 1997). When a person has an OI or cancer diagnosed clinically or by laboratory confirmation, he or she is regarded as having AIDS. The infections known as OIs are caused by organisms that exist in the environment of the body, such as on the skin, in the lungs, or in the gastrointestinal system; that remain latent until activated; and that become pathogenic when HIV has impaired the immunity system.

More than 20 different OIs and cancers have been associated with severe immune depletion. They include organisms from most biological categories of pathogens that can occur in our everyday environment. The range of complications arising from continued HIV infection varies from country to country, reflecting the differences in infectious agents that populations have encountered earlier in life or are reexposed to when immunosuppressed. In Western countries, the most common opportunistic diseases are cerebral toxoplasmosis, cryptococcal meningitis, cryptosporidium diarrhea, cytomegalovirus (CMV) retinitis, Kaposi's sarcoma, oesophageal candidiasis, and PCP (Bacellar and others 1994; Hoover and others 1993; Lanjewar and others 1996; Selik, Starcher, and Curran 1987). In Thailand and other resource-poor countries, because of the higher background incidence

**Table 3.3** Prevalence of Selected OIs in Australia, India, Thailand, the United States, and Zaire, 1998.
*percentage*

| Opportunistic infection | Australia | India | Thailand | United States | Zaire |
|---|---|---|---|---|---|
| Candidiasis | 30 | 40–60 | **40** | 13 | 25 |
| Cytomegalovirus | 30 | < 10 | **10** | 5 | 13 |
| Cryptococcus | 5–10 | 2–5 | **20** | 7 | 20 |
| Pneumocytosis carinii pneumonia | 30–50 | 2–5 | **15–20** | 65 | < 2% |
| Penicilliosis | Not seen | 5 | **5–25** | Not seen | Not seen |
| Toxoplasmosis | 10 | 2 | **5** | 5 | 10 |
| Tuberculosis | 3 | 45–65 | **30–40** | 3 | 40 |

*Source:* UNAIDS 1998.

of other infectious agents, cryptococcal meningitis, infectious diarrhea, nonspecific wasting syndrome (slim disease), toxoplasma encephalopathy, and TB are more commonly encountered (see table 3.3) (Beji and others 1994; Chacko and others 1995; Hira, Dupont, Lanjewar, and others 1998; Hira, Dupont, and Sirisanthana 1998; Sengupta, Lal, and Shrinivas 1994; Unnikrishnan and others 1993).

The time from AIDS diagnosis to death depends on the type of OI, the availability of care, and the adherence of the patient to prescribed prophylaxis and treatment. Assigning a specific timeframe to survival from diagnosis of AIDS is becoming less relevant as accessibility to ART increases. Nevertheless, primary prophylaxis for OIs remains one of the most important ongoing and successful strategies in response to care of patients with progressive HIV disease. In Thailand, until relatively recently, the perception was that inadequate recognition of the role of prophylaxis was common; less than 50 percent of HIV-positive patients cared for by the Thai Network of People Living with AIDS, a nongovernmental organization (NGO) were covered by PCP prophylaxis (Wilson and Ford 2004; World Bank 2000). Community groups mounted a concerted campaign to increase awareness of the low costs and clear benefits of PCP prophylaxis, so that by 2002 health services increased its use to more than 85 percent (Wilson and Ford 2004).

In addition to differences in the background prevalence of certain infections, differences in the level of immunosuppression required before an AIDS-defining illness occurs also vary within countries and populations. TB, which causes significant mortality in the population not infected by HIV, requires only moderate immune suppression before it can reactivate in previously exposed individuals. PCP usually occurs when CD4 cell counts have declined to below 200 cells per cubic millimeter, whereas CMV and atypical mycobacterial disease (mycobacterium avium complex, or MAC) usually arise when CD4 counts have dropped to below 50 cells per cubic millimeter (Selik, Starcher, and Curran 1987).

Starting ART in the presence of undiagnosed active TB may cause life-threatening complications because of immune reconstitution disease, which is expected to occur in up to 35 percent of patients who begin ART with a CD4 count of less than 50 cells per cubic millimeter. An important study from the Central Chest Hospital near Bangkok revealed disturbing information on HIV-TB coinfection (Punnotok and others 2000). In that study, conducted between 1995 and 1996, 2,587 newly registered patients with suspected pulmonary TB were considered for HIV screening. Of the 1,091 patients who had confirmed TB, the HIV prevalence was 22 percent. When those patients were compared with the HIV-negative TB patients, the authors found the HIV-TB patients were more likely to have isoniazid-resistant TB (10.9 percent compared with 3.5 percent) and multidrug-resistant TB (5.2 percent compared with 0.4 percent). That finding suggests that multidrug-resistant TB (MDR-TB) might develop among HIV-positive TB patients and then spread to HIV-negative people. Therefore, Thailand's policy of directly observed treatment of TB, which is designed to maximize adherence to TB treatment and to thus minimize the development of MDR-TB, is even more important for HIV-infected TB patients.

A common thought is that the differences in AIDS presentations in resource-poor countries, compared with Western countries, could be partially accounted for by few patients surviving their initial AIDS illnesses to become immunosuppressed enough to have reactivations of CMV or MAC. The widespread use of simple interventions, such as trimethoprim-sulfamethoxazole as PCP prophylaxis, has had a significant effect in delaying the onset of PCP, one of the most common initial AIDS-defining events, and has therefore positively influenced survival (Hoover and others 1993). However, prevention of PCP does not halt the relentless erosion of the immune system and prolongs life for only a short period. The only way to halt or delay progression of HIV disease is to interrupt viral replication, which is the aim of ART.

## Effect of ART on Survival

The time path that an HIV-infected person follows from initial infection to the first symptoms of the disease and then to death and the response of that person to treatment are known to be highly variable and to depend on a host of characteristics of the individual, the virus, the treatment regimen, and the social context. Less well known, but equally crucial for projecting the result of the treatment policy are the effects of such variables on the propensity of individuals to seek ART and to persist with treatment once it has begun. Appendix A summarizes the empirical information available at the time of writing on the relationship between those variables and disease progression, as well as on the somewhat technically complex process by which we have estimated these patterns given the available information and expert opinion. This section synthesizes that discussion for a less technical audience.

To make projections under specific policy alternatives, we adopt a simplified set of assumptions about seeking of treatment, persistence with treatment, and survival as influenced by three of the many variables:

- whether treatment begins relatively early (at CD4 counts between 50 and 200 cells per cubic millimeter or relatively late (at a CD4 count of 50 cells per cubic millimeter or below)

- whether the provision of care is augmented by the presence of an effective group of people living with HIV and AIDS (PHAs)

- whether the patient is on first-line therapy or on second-line therapy.[2]

The two panels of figure 3.2 display our characterization of the literature and the opinions of our clinical experts regarding the cumulative proportion of patients who leave a treatment regimen either by dropping out or, for patients on first-line therapy, by moving from first-line to second-line therapy. Panel (a) gives the patterns for the typical patient, who begins treatment late. Panel (b) gives the pattern for patients who begin early. Two of the four patterns within each panel display the assumed dropout pattern for individual patients receiving public sector ART on first-line or second-line therapy. The horizontal axis measures the time from the beginning of that type of

**Figure 3.2**  Persistence Assumptions for Patients Receiving Public and Augmented Public ART

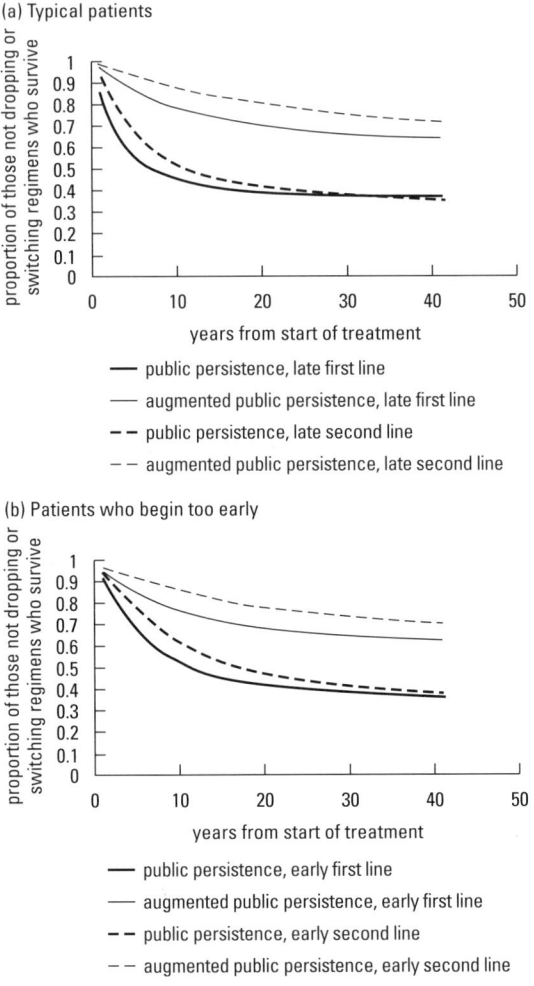

(a) Typical patients

years from start of treatment

— public persistence, late first line
— augmented public persistence, late first line
– – public persistence, late second line
– – augmented public persistence, late second line

(b) Patients who begin too early

years from start of treatment

— public persistence, early first line
— augmented public persistence, early first line
– – public persistence, early second line
– – augmented public persistence, early second line

*Source:* Authors.

care. Because the typical patient on second-line therapy would be starting after several years of first-line therapy, the less successful survival is partly explained by these extra years of sickness.

A survival curve can then be defined that is conditional on patients not dropping out of treatment or, for those on first-line therapy, not moving on to second-line therapy. The two panels of figure 3.3 display our assumptions regarding the conditional survival of patients who do not drop out or move on to second-line therapy. Panel (a) gives the survival patterns for patients who begin late, when their CD4 counts are 50 cells per cubic millimeter or below. Panel (b) gives the survival patterns for early starters. The four patterns within each panel give the assumptions for the two public modes of treatment and for first-line and second-line therapies. As for figure 3.2, the less successful survival of those on second-line therapy is partly explained by the extra years of sickness already spent on ineffective first-line therapy. The patterns clearly show the greater presumed success of public therapy when it is augmented by a supportive PHA group that facilitates patient adherence.

**Figure 3.3**  Survival Assumptions for Patients Receiving Public and Augmented Public ART

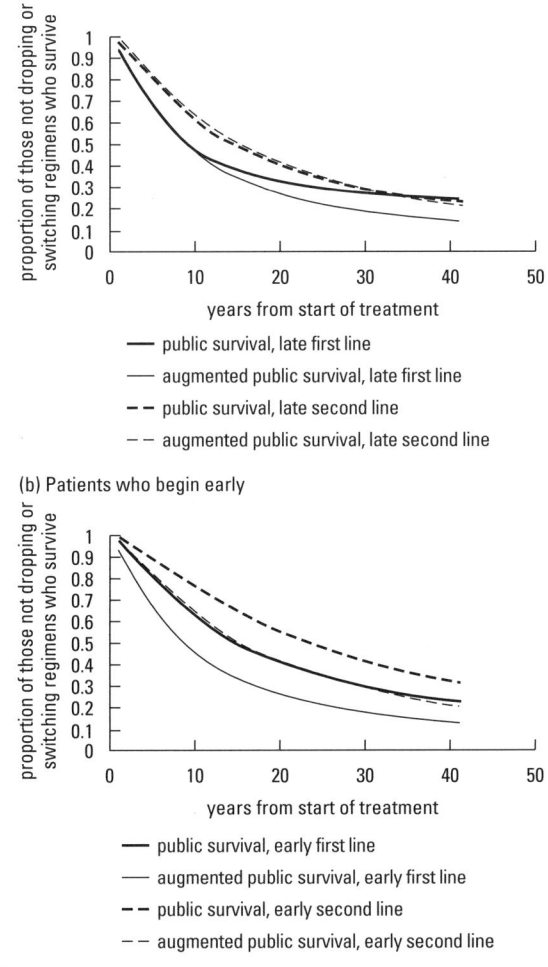

Source: Authors.

Patients who choose private sector care in Thailand are assumed to follow persistence and survival patterns identical to those that they would follow with augmented public care, hence obviating the need for the display of such patterns in the two figures. The report team believes that assumption is plausible because most private treatment in Thailand is of relatively high quality and because the patients who are willing and able to pay for private ART typically have the motivation and the social support to achieve high levels of adherence. Furthermore, in the face of growing competition from the augmented public system, private caregivers with low perceived success rates will fail to attract patients.

Because of the complexity of those options, direct computation does not easily yield an answer to this basic question: given the possibilities of dying, dropping out, or moving to second-line therapy, where the person might again drop out or die, what is the overall likely survival pattern of an individual who begins ART? The best way to derive such an answer is to use the Asian Epidemic Model (AEM) to assemble a pattern from all the possibilities. We do so by comparing the predictions of the AEM for our baseline—where there is very little ART—with the predictions from a specially constructed artificial scenario in which a single cohort of patients begins treatment in 2002, but new treatment starts revert to baseline levels in subsequent years. By comparing those two scenarios, we estimate the survival of the patients in that single 2002 cohort. Figure 3.4 presents the results.

**Figure 3.4** Survival of a Model Cohort of Patients across First-Line and Second-Line Treatment Regimens If They Are Recruited Early or Late

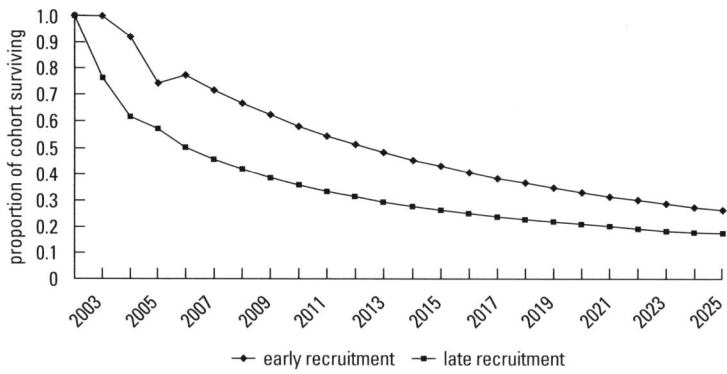

*Source:* Authors.

As expected from the inputs to the model, the survival experience is markedly better for patients recruited early when their CD4 counts are between 50 and 200 cells per cubic millimeter than when they are recruited late, when their CD4 counts are 50 cells per cubic millimeter or below. By truncating the survival curve at 2025, the 23rd year, one can estimate the mean survival time for early and late recruits. The mean *additional* survival, starting at the time of treatment initiation and compared with no ART, of early recruits is 10.3 years compared with 8.0 years for those patients recruited at the lower CD4 count. Thus, for every new patient recruited into ART, those years of life accrue to the individual and to society as a whole in the year of recruitment.

To interpret those numbers, we recall that patients who are recruited early would be typically 18 to 30 months from death, whereas those recruited late would be between 6 and 12 months away. Thus, early recruitment to ART is estimated to add 10.3 years to the 18 to 30 months that the person would have survived, and late recruitment is estimated to add 8.0 years to the person's life expectancy. Therefore, according to this model and the assumptions detailed earlier, a person who begins treatment two years early adds more than those two years to his or her life expectancy. If we set aside for a moment the issue of discounting and all costs other than the person's time, the investment of the two years of treatment appears to be worthwhile from the individual's perspective: two years of early treatment yields three or four years of extra life.

When we estimate the cost-effectiveness of ART policies, we will use those incremental life-years saved per person who begins treatment as an incidence-based measure of benefit. Because those streams of 10.3 life-years or 8.0 life-years saved extend over time, they must be converted to discounted life-years using the discount rate used in the analysis. For example, if all costs and benefits are discounted at 3 percent, then the number of incremental life-years saved per new patient on ART become 7.9 and 6.5 discounted life-years saved, respectively.

## Clinical Management of HIV Disease with ART

Management of ART is complex, and it requires not only significant capacity in terms of health service delivery, but also an accompanying range of counseling, testing, and laboratory services. Partly as a result of those requirements, scaling up ART treatment presents serious practical challenges. Challenges exist in any setting and even more so in environments where essential physical and human infrastructure may be lacking. The risk of providing ART without strict adherence to guidelines and agreed standards of care is the propagation of multidrug-resistant HIV. Nevertheless, the success of pilot studies in Africa and Brazil suggest that ART can be adequately delivered in resource-constrained settings and that rates of adherence to ART in poor countries may be as high as, or higher than, rates in resource-rich countries. In Thailand, with the advent of the single-tablet GPO-vir, NGOs are reporting much higher rates of adherence than previously obtained under multiple-tablet mono and dual therapy. Médecins sans Frontières (MSF) reports adherence of greater than 95 percent in a cohort of more than 400 patients who have had the benefit of a structured community support network (Wilson and Ford 2004). Similarly, a recent rapid assessment of adherence among PHAs on ART in Chiang Mai in northern Thailand, carried out by the Thai Ministry of Public Health (MOPH) and the Population Council, shows adherence rates of about 85 percent (Community Medicine Department, Chiang Mai University 2002).[3] Data from Siriraj University Hospital, however, suggest that good adherence cannot be automatically assumed: among 122 patients who started ART (with GPO-vir), only 60 percent were able to maintain an undetectable viral load after 12 months (Ratanasuwan 2004). The difference between the hospital's results and those obtained by MSF and in Chiang Mai may reflect the important role played by structured support networks and PHA peer groups in ensuring adherence. Interestingly, the Siriraj University Hospital adherence rate is similar to the rates expected in most cohorts in Western countries.

### Diagnosis of HIV and Recruitment of Patients into ART

The ideal paradigm for care of people with HIV is by diagnosis of HIV in its early stages, preferably while they are well and before they have an opportunity to transmit HIV to their children or their sexual partners or through blood-to-blood contact. Diagnosis should be accompanied by counseling about their personal and public health responsibilities. Patients should then be monitored regularly until they develop an HIV-related illness or experience a drop in their CD4 count below 200 cells per cubic millimeter, and they should start ART when they are adequately informed and have all necessary support systems to maximize adherence. Depending on the initial CD4 count, patients may need to be monitored only every six months. In Thailand, the current strategy of HIV diagnosis and recruitment of patients into ART is still working toward this ideal. Patients are generally diagnosed very late in their disease, when CD4 counts are well below 200 cells per cubic millimeter. The Thai Red Cross HIV/AIDS cohort, for example, reveals that 63 percent of attendees at the Anonymous Clinic between 1997 and 2003 had CD4 counts of less than 200 cells per cubic millimeter at the time of their HIV-positive diagnosis (table 3.4) (Duncombe 2004). Data from MOPH and MSF report similar findings. Late diagnosis and the ensuing need to start ART almost immediately could compound problems of poor adherence and could maximize the possibility of toxicity and of development of immune reconstitution disease.

Additional data on the predominantly late diagnosis of HIV are available from the January 2004 and January 2005 surveys of Thai clinicians (Gold and others 2005). Doctors were asked to estimate the proportion of their patients who commenced ART at a CD4 count of less than 50 cells per cubic millimeter. Irrespective of their sector of affiliation (private, public, university, or other), Thai doctors reported having a large proportion of patients commencing ART at CD4 counts of below 50 cells per cubic millimeter (figure 3.5).

Other data suggest that as treatment becomes more available and as HIV is more widely accepted in Thai society, people are seeking testing in the earlier stages of their HIV disease. Data from the Thai Red Cross Anonymous Clinic show progressively earlier diagnosis from 1997 to 2003 (table 3.5). The data are encouraging in suggesting that availability of treatment could be used to strengthen voluntary counseling and testing efforts.

**Table 3.4** Number of HIV-Positive Attendees at the Thai Red Cross Anonymous Clinic, Stratified by CD4 Cell Count, 1997–2003

| CD4 cell count (cells/mm³) | Number tested | Percentage of total |
| --- | --- | --- |
| < 100 | 6,655 | 41.3 |
| 100–200 | 3,554 | 22.0 |
| 200–350 | 3,133 | 19.4 |
| > 350 | 2,784 | 17.3 |
| Total | 16,126 | 100.0 |

*Source:* Duncombe 2004.

**Figure 3.5** Thai Doctors' Estimates of Patients Who Started ART with CD4 Counts of Less Than 50 Cells per cubic millimeter

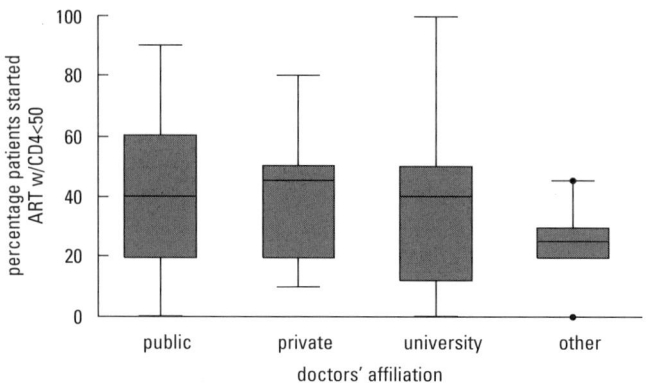

*Source:* Gold, Duncombe, and Masaki 2005.

**Table 3.5** Anonymous Clinic Attendees of Thai Red Cross Anonymous Clinic Whose CD4 Count Was Less Than 200 Cells per cubic millimeter, 1997–2003

| Year | Number of CD4 cell counts performed | Attendees with CD4 < 200 cells/mm³ (%) |
|------|------|------|
| 1997 | 341 | 79.5 |
| 1998 | 1,387 | 84.4 |
| 1999 | 2,712 | 88.1 |
| 2000 | 2,706 | 52.8 |
| 2001 | 2,505 | 64.2 |
| 2002 | 3,194 | 55.9 |
| 2003[a] | 3,281 | 55.0 |
| Overall | 16,126 | 63.3 |

*Source:* Duncombe 2004.
a. Up to December 18.

To assess the importance of early diagnosis, one can compare the costs of care for patients who start ART while their immune function is still competent with the costs of care for those who start very late, as occurs throughout Thailand. Some indication may be gained from a recent Canadian study (Krentz, Auld, and Gill 2004). In that study, the authors compared a range of hospital and treatment costs for patients who presented for care at a CD4 count of less than 200 cells per cubic millimeter with costs for those patients who presented with a CD4 count of greater than 200 cells per cubic millimeter. Patients who presented with a CD4 count of less than 100 cells per cubic millimeter incurred almost three times the additional costs compared with those patients with CD4 counts greater than 200 cells per cubic millimeter. Such costs were mainly attributed to hospitalizations and treatment for OIs before starting ART. This finding is confirmed for Thailand by a recent study that found that patients with CD4 counts of less than 50 cells per cubic millimeter at their first outpatient visit incurred costs on average 30 percent higher than those with CD4 counts of more than 200 cells per cubic millimeter (B 37,190 per year compared with B 28,986 per year) (Supakakunti and others 2004).

### Clinical Challenges at Initiation of ART

Like all medications, ART has a range of potential toxicities that can vary from mildly irritating to life threatening. Although individual and class-specific toxicities are known, difficulties arise in trying to predict exactly which patient will develop toxicities and when and how that patient will respond to treatment of those adverse reactions. Drug toxicities compromise the benefits of ART, both in inducing potentially serious health problems and in reducing the chances of a patient remaining on therapy. Those effects can be considered either acute or chronic events. One must recognize that because of the differences in toxicities that may manifest within an individual, one drug from a particular class may be inappropriate, yet another drug from the same class may be well tolerated (Duncombe 2004; Gold and others 2005).

Concerns about the long-term development of drug toxicities have prompted medical authorities in many countries, including Thailand, to adopt a conservative approach to ART. Recent guidelines recommend ART for only those individuals in whom the risk of disease progression is greater than the possible drug-related concerns (Carpenter and others 2000). The following information on when and how to start ART is based on the National Guidelines for the Clinical Management of HIV Infection in Children and Adults (MOPH 2002).

#### When to Start?
The enrollment criteria for adults are as follows:

- AIDS

- Symptomatic HIV disease with or without a CD4 count of less than 250 cells per cubic millimeter (CDC clinical B or C)

- Asymptomatic HIV with CD4 count of less than 200 cells per cubic millimeter.

For children, the following enrollment criteria apply:

• All children less than 12 years old

• Children age 12 years or older with World Health Organization (WHO) clinical stage B and C or a CD4 count of less than 200 cells per cubic millimeter.

*How to Start?*

The recommended first-line antiretroviral regimen in Thailand is the fixed-dose combination of lamivudine, stavudine, and nevirapine, produced and sold by the Government Pharmaceutical Office (GPO) as GPO-vir.[4] In addition, the MOPH has defined two alternative regimens for those patients who develop intolerance to one of the GPO-vir components. The three available first-line regimens under the National Access to Antiretroviral Program for People Living with HIV and AIDS (NAPHA) are as follows:

• stavudine + lamivudine + nevirapine (GPO-vir)

• stavudine + lamivudine + efavirenz

• stavudine + lamivudine + indinavir/ritonavir.

Some 80 percent of patients are estimated to be taking the first regimen, while an estimated 15 percent are taking the second regimen and an estimated 5 percent will eventually have to be moved to the third regimen.

The efficacy, safety, and tolerability of the GPO-vir combination in patients who are taking ART for the first time were recently evaluated by the multicountry 2NN study (van Leth and others 2004).[5] The 2NN study was a randomized comparative open-label trial of first-line ART with regimens containing nevirapine, efavirenz, or both drugs combined in addition to stavudine and lamivudine in a treatment-naive population. The characteristics of the population of patients in the 2NN study are similar to the population requiring ART in Thailand. The study enrolled 1,216 ART-naive participants in 17 countries, with 200 enrolled at the HIV Netherlands Australia Thailand Research Collaboration (HIV-NAT) at the Thai Red Cross AIDS Research Centre in Bangkok. Among those participants, 607 were randomized to receive stavudine (40 milligrams twice daily if bodyweight is greater than 60 kilograms and 30 milligrams twice daily

## Box 3.1 Key Challenges for Second-Line ART in Thailand

MOPH's second-line protocol is summarized as follows:

- failure based on drop of CD4 of more than 30 percent (immunological failure) or on occurrence of an OI after two years on ART (clinical failure)
- viral-load testing once per year (virological failure)
- resistance testing if viral load is greater than 5,000 copies per milliliter
- three alternative regimens:
  - didanosine+ lamivudine + idinavir/ritonavir
  - didanosine + lamivudine + lopinavir/ritonavir
  - lopinavir/ritonavir + saquinavir.

However, the existing protocol of second-line regimens in Thailand faces key challenges for successful implementation of ART because of late diagnosis of treatment failure, cross-resistance to many nucleoside reverse transcriptase inhibitor drugs, limited efficacy, and high costs of drugs. Thus, Thailand must investigate other policy options that lead to effective and sustainable implementation of the ART program.

### Treatment Failure

Treatment failure can be detected in three ways:

- *Virological failure.* The patient's viral load becomes undetectable after ART begins, but later becomes detectable and generally increases over time. The cutoff of viral-load level that the doctor might use as a reason to change to a second-line regimen is not standard but depends on several factors, such as availability and cost of second-line drugs, the rate of rise of viral load, and the rate of decline of CD4 count.
- *Immunological failure.* This failure happens later than virological failure. After the level of HIV in the body has risen for some time, the CD4 count will fall. More than one definition of immunological failure exists: the WHO requires a fall of 50 percent and the MOPH requires a fall of 30 percent. Another problem is that the daily measurement of CD4 level is affected by many factors, such as concurrent infections.
- *Clinical failure.* Later still, after the CD4 count has fallen to low levels, the patient will develop an OI and become sick.

Thus, depending on how failure is diagnosed and how the criteria is used to make the diagnosis, failure may be early or late.

### Resistance

At the start of the process of failure, HIV will probably be resistant to only one of the ARV drugs in the first-line regimen. Later, resistance may occur to the other drugs. In late failure, HIV will often be cross-resistant to other drugs of the same class that the patient has never taken. However, cross-resistance does not occur across different classes of drugs, only within each class. Many kinds of resistance exist, and in each class of drug, cross-resistance occurs at different rates and levels.

---

**Box 3.1    Continued**

*Monitoring and Testing*

Compared with the past, enhanced possibility now exists to diagnose failure of first-line treatment. Such diagnosis is possible because of the increased availability and capacity of testing and monitoring of ART treatment, particularly through

- wider availability and lower cost of viral-load tests
- wider availability of HIV-resistance testing.

  MOPH has introduced viral-load testing and a limited range of second-line anti-retroviral drug regimens into the national treatment program.

*Cost of Second-Line ART*

The cost of a second-line treatment program remains extremely high and also depends on many factors:

- price of testing (reagents and other costs) for viral load and resistance
- early or late diagnosis of failure, thus allowing a determination of which second-line drugs are likely to be effective
- number of patients whose failure was diagnosed clinically, immunologically, or virologically
- cutoff of viral load used for diagnosing failure
- price of the second-line drugs and availability of generic drugs or low-cost branded drugs.

---

if bodyweight is less than 60 kilograms), lamivudine (150 milligrams twice daily), and nevirapine (200 milligrams twice daily). Of the 607 participants randomized to this group, 387 were available for the first 48-week analysis. That analysis showed that 65.4 percent of those participating had a viral load of less than 50 copies per milliliter after one year of treatment with stavudine, lamivudine, and nevirapine. A moderate or severe rash associated with nevirapine was reported in 3.6 percent of the participants. Moderate or severe liver toxicity was reported in 7.8 percent of the participants. In the first 48 weeks of therapy, 22 percent of the participants changed ART.

*Immune Reconstitution Syndrome*
One of the challenges posed by late diagnosis of HIV and late commencement of ART is the increased risk of immune reconstitution syndrome (IRS). Restoration of immune function with ART can have

adverse consequences that may be confused with toxicity related directly to ART. IRS is caused by augmented immune responses to pathogens that are already present, but the mechanism is poorly understood. The incidence of IRS can be as high as 30 to 40 percent and is related to the degree of immune depletion present at the time of commencing ART. The most common IRS reactions are to cryptococcal infections and TB, and most occur within the first month of starting ART. IRS can also occur with most other OIs, including CMV, where patients may develop an immune recovery vitritis as many as eight months after commencing ART. The MSF experience with patients who begin ART when their CD4 count is greater than 50 cells per cubic millimeter is that up to 17 percent may die of AIDS-related complications, including IRS, within the first several months.[6] In some centers, like Siriraj University Hospital in Bangkok, the approach to preventing IRS is to screen patients for OIs before they start ART. That screening process is appealing, but it can be expensive and is only practical only in major teaching hospital facilities. The most feasible option for ameliorating the effect of IRS is to encourage people to engage voluntary counseling and testing (VCT) services earlier in their illness and to begin ART when their CD4 count is about 200 cells per cubic millimeter.

### Adherence to and Maximizing of the Benefits of ART

Treatment adherence or compliance broadly means the extent to which the patient follows medical instructions in taking his or her medications. It means taking the correct dosage, taking it the correct way, and taking it every time. Adherence is more difficult to maintain when medications need to be taken according to a precise schedule on a long-term basis, as is the case for many chronic illnesses, including HIV/AIDS. Those HIV medications that need to be taken on a long-term basis include ARTs, prophylactic medications for prevention of OIs, and medications for treatment of OIs (particularly TB). Maintenance of almost perfect adherence to ART is probably the most important determinant of success or failure of treatment.

Incontrovertible data suggest that adherence is one of the strongest predictors of CD4 count response to ART and therefore the best parameter of success. Wood and others (2004) evaluated the response of 1,522 ART-naive patients who were stratified by CD4 count and by subsequent adherence. The investigators stratified patients according

## Box 3.2    Pediatric HIV/AIDS in Thailand

In 1991, the first pediatric HIV case was identified in Thailand. As of the end of 2005, about 42,000 cumulative cases of children with HIV infection were reported. Thailand has received international recognition for its effort in preventing mother-to-child transmission of HIV. A recent evaluation found that of 573,600 women who gave birth, 92 to 98 percent received prenatal care and 93.3 percent were tested for HIV. Of the 6,646 women who were found to be HIV positive, more than 90 percent received pre-natal care and, of those, 4,659 (70.1 percent) received ART before delivery to prevent HIV transmission. Of the 6,475 infants born to the HIV-positive mothers, 5,741 (88.7 percent) received prophylactic ART. The number of new cases of infants with HIV infection in 2002 was between 600 and 800, down from almost 5,000 in 1998. Despite this impressive response, an estimated 25,000 children currently are living with HIV/AIDS, and at least one-half of them require ART to ameliorate the onset of severe HIV disease. The treatment of children with ART, as part of the MOPH Access to Care (ATC) initiative, began in 1998 with 800 children and was expanded to 2,000 children in 2000. Currently, all eligible children should have access to ART in Thailand.

Many complex issues arise in treating HIV-infected children, not the least of which is that one or both of their parents may already have died of AIDS. An estimated 300,000 AIDS orphans live in Thailand, so both HIV-infected and non-HIV-infected children may be living with grandparents, other relatives, or friends. These caretakers may not have sufficient time to ensure appropriate adherence to ART and management of toxicities and intercurrent infections for the HIV-infected children while still arranging for the needs and supervision of all the children in their care. Moreover, the impact of HIV disease on children goes beyond the range of OIs usually described in adults. Clear evidence demonstrates that HIV-infected children have significantly higher rates of psychiatric illness, especially depression and behavioral disorders, compared with their peers. Those problems will also affect their ability to take and adhere to ART. In Thailand, the outcomes of children on ART are, in general, parallel to those of adults.

Because most HIV-infected children will be diagnosed soon after birth, therapy should commence at the most opportune time. However, considerable international debate exists as to the best time to start ART and as to the most appropriate regimen. Some early data also suggest that, with careful monitoring, it may be possible to reduce ART toxicities by structured treatment interruptions in children with no loss of ART efficacy. The prevalence of known metabolic and physical (fat redistribution) toxicities associated with ART is as high in children as in adults. Moreover, other problems not prevalent in adults, such as bone mineral density abnormalities, for example, osteopenia (53 percent) and the more serious osteoporosis (23 percent) were observed in a cohort of children on ART in Texas.

The Thai network of clinical research in pediatric HIV/AIDS includes HIV-NAT and centers at Chulalongkorn University Hospital, Khon Kaen University, and Queen Sirikit National Institute of Child Health. HIV-NAT currently has initiated six pediatric studies, and five more are planned. HIV-NAT commenced its first pediatric study (HIV-NAT 010) in November 2001. That was a pilot study was designed to evaluate when to start ART in HIV-infected children. Children with mild or moderate symptoms and with a CD4 cell count between 15 and 24 percent (moderate immune suppression) were randomized to start ART (GPO-vir) immediately or to wait until their CD4 count fell below 15 percent. That study enrolled 43 children at HIV-NAT and at Khon Kaen University. A study involving 300 children was proposed for 2004. HIV-NAT also follows 60 children who are being treated with highly active antiretroviral therapy (HAART) based on nonnucleoside reverse transcriptase inhibitors (NNRTIs) through the ATC program. Those patients are mainly older children with low CD4 counts who previously had no access to ART because of financial difficulties. In each of the past six months, approximately four new cases have appeared.

A cross-sectional study of genotypic resistance in 100 children treated with nucleoside reverse transcriptase inhibitors (NRTIs) was undertaken at HIV-NAT and Queen Sirikit National Institute of Child Health. The preliminary results show that a majority of children harbor reverse transcriptase mutations. In Thailand, until recently, dual NRTI has been the main ART regimen used. The results of that study will help providers to plan for salvage therapy in those children. HIV-NAT has also initiated two pharmacokinetic studies to find the ideal dosing of the following protease inhibitors in children. One study examines lopinavir/ritonavir + saquinavir, and the other study examines nelfinavir. Those studies are important because the correct dosages in children are not known. The lopinavir/ritonavir + saquinavir combination is a potential salvage regimen for children with resistance to the most widely used HAART in Thailand, GPO-vir.

HIV-NAT understands the importance of addressing psychosocial issues in children and families affected by HIV. HIV-NAT works closely with the Wednesday Friends Club, a peer support group of the Thai Red Cross AIDS Research Centre, to counsel caregivers. At each clinic, representatives from the Wednesday Friends Club hold individual and group counseling sessions with caregivers while the children play and listen to stories. HIV-NAT is exploring two main issues:

- the factors that affect adherence to ART and
- the reasons behind caregivers' decisions not to disclose to children their HIV diagnosis.

An added benefit of HIV-NAT pediatric studies is the opportunity to identify HIV-infected parents who have not sought care. Almost all of those parents now receive ART if appropriate. Clinical care is provided through HIV-NAT's adult clinical trials and ATC programs. In 2004, HIV-NAT planned to launch five new pediatric studies:

- a pharmacokinetic study of an investigational ART
- a structured treatment-interruption study
- a prospective cohort of 300 children on NNRTI-based HAART with seven sites in Thailand
- a salvage therapy study for children failing dual NRTIs
- the full study (following HIV-NAT 010) of immediate versus deferred ART initiation.

*Source:* Gold and others 2004.

to their CD4 count on initiation of ART. The time to record a rise of at least 50 cells per cubic millimeter was used as an indicator of response to therapy. Response was determined during each of five 15-week periods after therapy began. Adherence was calculated as the amount of medication required for perfect adherence divided by the actual amount of medication dispensed to each patient during the first year of treatment. The investigators used a cutoff level of 75 percent adherence as the indicator of adequate or inadequate adherence. Irrespective of the ART drugs used, statistically significant improvements in CD4 counts were seen between adherent and nonadherent patient groups at all strata of baseline CD4 counts. The investigators also conducted a univariate analysis for predictors of CD4 count response and found that male gender, increasing age, adherence, injecting drug use, and baseline HIV RNA were all significantly associated with CD4 cell response. In a subsequent multivariate analysis that controlled for those factors, male gender, adherence, protease inhibitor use, and baseline HIV RNA were all associated with a response (table 3.6).

A particularly important finding for the Thai situation was the relationship between baseline CD4 count, adherence, and response rate. The investigators conducted a more detailed analysis in which they looked at patients who had adherence of greater than 95 percent compared with the 75 to 95 percent group. They found a significant difference in the response rate at 24 months for patients who were 95 percent adherent (72.8 percent responsive) compared with the second strata, where the response rate was only 50.7 percent. Those observations indicate that considerable attention must be directed at the adherence of patients who begin ART at late stages of HIV disease in order to achieve the maximum benefit of therapy. The observations further reinforce the notion that it is never too late to begin therapy

**Table 3.6** CD4 Count and Interquartile Range at the Fifth 15-week Follow-up Compared with the Baseline

| | CD4 count (Interquartile range) | | |
| | Adherent | Nonadherent | |
| Baseline CD4 count | | | p Value |
| --- | --- | --- | --- |
| < 50 | 200 (130–290) | 60 (10–30) | p = 0.009 |
| 50–199 | 300 (180–390) | 125 (40–210) | p < 0.001 |
| > 200 | 550 (410–720) | 300 (250–505) | p < 0.001 |

*Source:* Adapted from Woods and others 2004. Interquartile ranges are from Duncombe and others 2004.

and that substantial gains in CD4 counts can be achieved with excellent adherence. In that study, 39 percent of the patients presented with a CD4 count of less than 200 cells per cubic millimeter. The conclusion is that any triple combination ART will achieve significant patient benefit, if the therapy is taken as directed. One should note that all care for patients in that study was provided free of any charge.

Despite the advent of a reduced pill burden compared with five years ago, as well as less frequent dosing, adherence in HIV patients in developed countries is far from optimal, with most studies indicating a long-term adherence rate of less than 60 percent in community-based studies, as compared with the controlled and supported situation found in clinical trials. No strong evidence exists to suggest that people in resource-poor countries will adhere less to ART than their counterparts in resource-rich countries. Factors that appear to positively affect adherence in resource-rich country settings include the frequency of outpatient visits, education, age, and lifestyle factors (no alcohol or recreational drug use) (Kleeberger and others 2004). No comparable statistical research to date examines what factors affect adherence in Thailand. However, some qualitative evidence drawn from interviews and focus groups with PHAs does exist (box 3.3). From the perspective of PHAs, the medical and emotional side effects of ART and the lack of support and sufficient information about ART are major factors decreasing adherence. Lack of reliability in drug supply is also mentioned, as are financial costs.

One must also understand what providers feel are the determinants of good adherence. Table 3.7 reports the factors that respondents to the HIV-NAT Survey of Thai Physicians regarded as important in adherence to ART.

Increasing the effectiveness of interventions to improve adherence may have far greater effect on the health of the population than any improvement in specific medical treatments. The WHO reports that studies consistently find significant cost savings and increases in the effectiveness of health interventions that are attributable to low-cost interventions for improving adherence.

### Development of Resistance and Its Effect on the Use of ART

Resistance to ARTs is probably the greatest threat to the control of HIV. As each new therapy is released and tested in the community,

**Box 3.3   Behavioral Aspects of Adherence to ART in Thailand Based on Results from Interviews and Focus Groups with PHAs**

*Aim*

This study assessed qualitative information from PHAs on their experience of accessing ART through the MOPH system and on their experience in taking ART, with the aim of determining factors than affect adherence and quality of life. In addition, the study was designed to record individual stories about their experience with the health care system as related to care and treatment.

*Methodology*

Using an open format, interviews and focus group discussions were conducted by Dr. Seri Phongphit with PHAs from Bangkok, Khon Kaen, and Suratthani. Students and staff from Chiang Mai University, Khon Kaen University, and Rajabhat Institute assisted with recording the responses at workshops and meetings.

*Results*

Because information was qualitative and subjective, it is appropriate to present it in narrative form. The general impressions can be summarized as follows:

- *Factors that improve adherence.* PHAs have an overwhelming feeling that wider availability of ART has given them hope where previously there was none. They are now able to plan for the future and to take care of their families by continuing to work. Because PHAs can now live a more normal life, they feel less stigma and discrimination. They feel they are less of a burden on society and are more accepted by their communities. Because many PHAs have seen their friends and family members die of AIDS, they believe that ART is a key to their continuing survival. The presence of community support networks is vital in providing stability to and continuity in taking ART. Education of family members is also important because they need to understand the rigorous effort required to take ART. The availability of ART through the public hospital system is important because it reduces the cost of ART, even though PHAs may still have to pay for monitoring tests.
- *Factors that impede adherence.* PHAs believe that when they start ART, they are not given enough information by prescribing doctors and the public health

resistant strains are identified that can result in either partial or complete drug resistance, depending on the particular genomic mutation. In countries where ART has been available for more than a decade, most HIV present in the community has at least one resistant mutation. The major underlying causes for drug resistance, which leads to

system, in general, about the side effects of ART, especially the immediate problems of nausea, diarrhea, change in mood, and rash, as well as the long-term issues of facial wasting and weight gain. Those side effects will encourage people to stop ART because many believe that ART is a cure, rather than needing to be taken on an ongoing basis. PHAs have the impression that the health care system imposes many lifestyle restrictions on them in order to be eligible for subsidized ART. They are told to avoid drinking alcohol, smoking, having children, and disclosing their HIV status to anyone, which is clearly an individual perception and not seen as universal in Thailand. Because they are diagnosed with HIV so late in their illness, PHAs feel that they need to start ART immediately and that they have no time to prepare socially and mentally for the commitment to taking ART. The "30-Baht" scheme provides considerable benefits, but it is not portable. Therefore, PHAs cannot access ART at hospitals outside their area of residence. Hospitals are usually visited as a last resort when PHAs are already ill. Because most voluntary counseling and testing services are located within the public hospital facility, they are not used early in HIV infection.

Opinions of numerous patients and doctors regarding factors that affect adherence have been gathered from the HIV-NAT conference survey and are shown in table 3.6. When we compare these opinions, we note a number of commonalities:

- improved education and information for patients, their family members, and health care workers
- subsidized HIV testing and monitoring to encourage patients to be tested earlier in their disease and to reduce the cost burden of treatment with ART
- community information programs to lessen the fear of HIV and to reduce stigma and discrimination
- government support for community support groups that provide essential support to help patients remain on ART

This behavioral survey underlines the fact that GPO-vir is an effective, relatively low-cost and low-toxicity treatment for HIV/AIDS, compared with the more toxic and expensive alternatives. It is essential that the health care system, at all levels, work with patients and the community to keep as many people on this therapy for as long as possible.

*Source:* Phongphit 2004.

treatment failure, are poor adherence, poor absorption, inadequate potency of the regimen, and drug-to-drug interaction that results in lowered blood levels. Resistant mutations develop simply because of Darwinian selection: if the drug level in plasma or cells is not high enough to suppress viral replication, then mutant strains will survive,

**Table 3.7** Clinician Opinions on Reasons for Poor Adherence to ART
*percentage*

| Reasons for poor adherence | Very important | Important | Not important |
|---|---|---|---|
| Financial difficulties | 78.1 | 18.3 | 3.7 |
| Medical side effects | 53.7 | 42.7 | 3.7 |
| Lifestyle factors | 47.6 | 42.7 | 9.8 |
| Social difficulties | 45.7 | 48.2 | 6.2 |
| Psychological difficulties | 37.8 | 52.4 | 9.8 |
| Illness associated with HIV | 34.2 | 61.0 | 4.9 |
| Medication factors | 34.2 | 58.5 | 7.3 |
| Concerns about confidentiality | 30.5 | 56.1 | 13.4 |
| Beliefs about effectiveness of treatment | 29.3 | 43.9 | 26.8 |
| Misunderstanding about need to take long term | 26.8 | 62.2 | 11.0 |
| Patient uncertainty about ability to adhere | 23.5 | 63.0 | 13.6 |
| Beliefs about HIV | 19.5 | 69.5 | 11.0 |
| Drug use | 19.2 | 50.0 | 30.8 |
| Alcohol use | 17.5 | 46.3 | 36.3 |
| Cultural belief | 14.6 | 56.1 | 29.3 |
| Beliefs about Western medicine | 11.1 | 51.9 | 37.0 |

*Source:* Gold, Duncombe, and Masaki, 2004 and 2005
*Note:* Because of rounding, percentages may not total to 100.0 percent.

which are then selected for their drug-resistant capacity. Two types of resistance are measured:

• genotype, which determines the genetic sequencing of the viral genome and describes whether specific mutations that have been observed to confer resistance are present

• phenotype, which determines the susceptibility of viral culture to different concentrations of a drug.

When those measurements are taken together, they can provide a valuable guide to the potential efficacy of different drug concentrations. Unfortunately, the technology required to perform those tests is expensive (up to US$600 per test) (B 24,000) and requires sophisticated laboratory support that is impractical to achieve in most settings. Resistance testing is not required to manage HIV appropriately because it is well accepted that monotherapy with any of the ART drugs will result in rapid development of resistance, as will adherence of less than about 95 percent, irrespective of the ART combinations chosen. Authorities have argued that anything less than triple therapy will be ineffective in managing patients on ART because development of resistance is inevitable. However, in a recent retrospective cohort study at Lampang Hospital in northern Thailand, patients who were treated with dual therapy had a clear advantage in survival over patients who were treated with monotherapy or patients who received no ART at all. The effect of ART on mortality was quantified by using a hazard ratio, after adjusting for sex, age group, year of registration, clinical status at first visit, and CD4 count group. The adjusted hazard ratio of monotherapy to no therapy was 0.65 and to dual therapy was 0.43. Those ratios suggest that even a suboptimum ART regimen can have substantial survival benefits.

Between the inexpensive CD4 tests and the expensive genetic sequencing tests lie the viral-load tests, which currently cost B3,000 to B5,000 (US$75–125) per test in Thailand. Because treatment failure in a patient often reveals itself as an increase in viral load before the CD4 count declines or OIs appear, viral-load tests are a useful signal to the clinician that it is time to switch the patient to second-line therapy. By switching therapies as soon as viral load begins to climb, the patient may avoid cross-resistance problems and thus have more success on second-line therapy. Therefore, incorporating viral-load tests into the cost of first-line therapy is justified if second-line therapy is available, but not otherwise.[7]

### Community- and NGO-Based Support to Enhance Adherence

The supportive role of community in HIV care is a fundamental aspect of the Thai response to the HIV/AIDS epidemic. Community-based organizations have been involved in providing home-based and palliative care since the early days of the epidemic. That role has now expanded to supporting patients on ART and providing their family members with the necessary knowledge to enhance the patients' adherence. Preliminary data suggest much higher rates of adherence to ART when adequate support networks are in place. NGOs and community-based organizations are the main vehicles for such support. Box 3.5 gives examples of NGO and community-involvement in support and care of PHAs in Thailand.

**Box 3.4    Can Direct Observed Therapy Strategies Be Applied to Provide More Effective ART?**

HIV management with ART is almost unique in medicine. It requires mostly young patients to take complex regimens over long periods with no respite and to maintain a minimum of 95 percent adherence. In the case of TB, for example, where similar regimens are taken for only some months, poor adherence led to a sweeping epidemic of multidrug-resistant TB (MDR-TB) that could only be prevented by introducing comprehensive directly observed treatment short course (DOTS) program. Although considering the use of DOTS for HIV is appealing, the long-term nature of treatment and the stigma attached to HIV disease are significant obstacles to this approach. Nevertheless, support is growing in international programs to use DOTS to expand ART. Evidence from small community-based treatment programs in Haiti, for example, suggest that DOTS with ART can be delivered effectively in poor settings if there is an uninterrupted supply of high-quality drugs (Farmer and others 2001a, 2001b).

In Thailand, this approach is gaining some currency, and with integration of the TB and HIV portfolios within MOPH, pilot studies will likely be used to test that strategy. The overlapping problems of HIV and TB are well known in Thailand, where TB represents about 40 percent of OIs. Following the rise of MDR-TB throughout Thailand, the MOPH strengthened the DOTS, which is now widespread and well accepted. The concept of using this process to provide lifelong therapy is appealing but not without problems. On the positive side, enabling TB and HIV therapy to be given simultaneously would allow the most efficient use of limited resources. Because HIV/TB coinfected patients have a higher mortality rate than patients with TB alone, integration of therapy would reduce TB mortality rates. Integration of services may also reduce the stigma and discrimination felt by patients who are treated for HIV and TB separately and by different management strategies. However, a range of potentially negative consequences of integration also can occur. TB therapy usually consists of several drugs given twice a day, albeit with a limited time of treatment. The additional HIV drugs, with their own side effects and immune reconstitution problems, may have a negative impact on both programs. In addition, there are important drug interactions between HIV and TB therapies, although the WHO has introduced recommendations to adjust the dosage of efavirenz when used with rifampin-containing regimens. The incidence of immune reconstitution disease has been observed to be as high as 36 percent in patients with HIV/TB when they start on ART, which complicates early patient care because it may be impossible to distinguish this problem from the side effects of ART or the TB medication or from the appearance of new disease manifestations. In that regard, training and support of health care workers to provide appropriate standards of patient care is very challenging. Provision of HIV management through the TB DOTS network remains an appealing but unproven strategy to improve efficiency and enhance adherence. Thailand is in an ideal position to establish research projects to test this strategy in community-based settings where high levels of donor support are not used to affect outcomes.

### Box 3.5  The Effect of a Comprehensive Care Program for PHA, Supported by MSF, in Ban Laem District Hospital

Ban Laem Hospital, 150 kilometers south of Bangkok in Petchburi province, is a 30 bed hospital serving a population of 45,000 people. In 2003, HIV prevalence in pregnant women in the region was 1.5 percent. In 1996, a senior nurse with a special interest in bereavement counseling set up a support group for relatives of patients who had died. As it happened, the three people who attended regularly were HIV-positive women whose husbands had died of AIDS. The group developed into a PHA peer support group; was named *Tan Tanod* (meaning palm sugar, a local product); and was formally launched in 1998 with a permanent meeting room in the hospital and with funding from the local government. At the request of the hospital, MSF provided training on health care and ongoing technical support for both hospital staff and PHAs. Tan Tanod currently has 114 members.

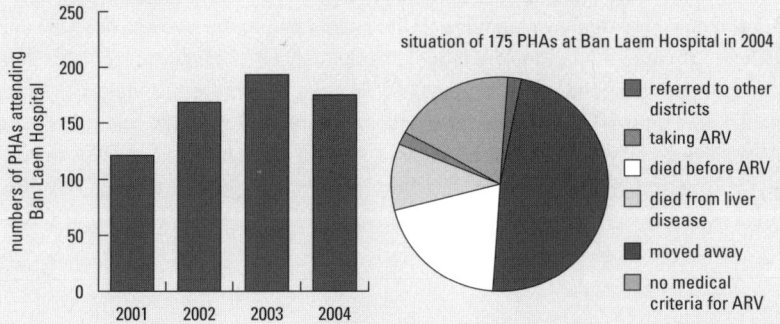

The antiretroviral (ARV) drug project in Ban Laem was launched in October 2001 with a 10-person project committee comprising four hospital staff members, four PHAs, and two MSF staff members. An HIV clinic was set up, initially on one day per week. In 2001, 120 PHAs visited the hospital for treatment. Soon after ARV drugs became available in the hospital, the number of PHAs visiting the hospital increased. The hospital has since moved from the concept of an ARV drug project with a limited quota of patients to the concept that AIDS is like other diseases, and all patients with clinical indications are treated with ARV drugs. Clinic days increased to twice weekly when the number of patients on ARV drugs increased beyond 75. Home visits are done three days per week—by PHAs on two days per week and jointly by PHAs and a nurse on the remaining day. In 2003, the hospital installed two condom vending machines; two condoms are dispensed for B 5 (US$0.12).

During 2004, 175 PHAs visited the hospital for treatment. Among those PHAs, 4 came from other districts and were referred to their local hospital; 86 (49 percent) now take ARV drugs; 32 (18 percent) died before ARV drugs were initiated; and 13 (7 percent)—all with very low CD4 counts—died of OIs within two months of starting ARV drugs. One has since died of end-stage liver disease, and three others have moved to

**Box 3.5 Continued**

other districts. Thirty-six (21 percent) do not fulfill medical criteria to begin use of ARV drugs because they are asymptomatic and their CD4 count is above 250: all of these patients are women diagnosed as HIV positive during pregnancy or their male partners. Of the 120 PHAs who visited the hospital during 2001 before the ARV drug project began, 87 (79 percent) required admission and 30 (25 percent) died. By 2004, the admission rate had fallen to 22 percent, and the death rate to 8 percent. The death rate of 25 percent in 2001 was linked with the correct treatment of OIs in the hospital and the existence of a home care program; the death rate would probably have been higher in the absence of these factors. The reason that the death rate has fallen from only 25 percent to 8 percent is that most PHAs do not visit a hospital until they are already sick with advanced immune suppression: in patients taking ARV drugs, the median CD4 count at the time of initiation of ARV drugs was 26 cells per $mm^3$.

After taking ARV drugs for one year, the leader of Tan Tanod became pregnant in 2003 and delivered healthy twin boys, to the delight of both herself and her husband. The new PHA leader (also on ARV drugs) has recently been employed by the hospital as a night guard, a good indication that AIDS is regarded in this hospital as a normal disease. It is unusual in Thailand for a hospital to give a leadership role to a known HIV-positive employee, in particular one who is open about his HIV status in the community. Other district hospitals in Petchburi province provide ARV drugs. The Thai

## Effect of ART on HIV Transmission

Public policy makers need to consider not only the direct effects of ART policy on the patients receiving ART, but also the indirect effects of ART on the creation of new cases of HIV infection.[8] Increasing evidence exists, for example, that the availability of ART may lead to complacency and increased risk behavior by people on ART and to negative and positive aspects of HIV in surrounding communities. (Dukers and others 2001; Stolte and others 2001; Van de Ven and others 2005). Assessing those spillover effects of ART on people other than the patients is an indispensable part of designing policy. Table 3.8 provides a classification of those indirect, or external, effects into biological and behavioral effects on transmission. Within each of the categories, the effects could be beneficial, by slowing transmission, or adverse, by accelerating it.

Network of PHA groups, MSF, and the provincial health department are working together to establish and strengthen PHA groups in the neighboring hospitals. One hopes that these groups can provide practical support for PHA benefiting from the wider access to ARV drugs.

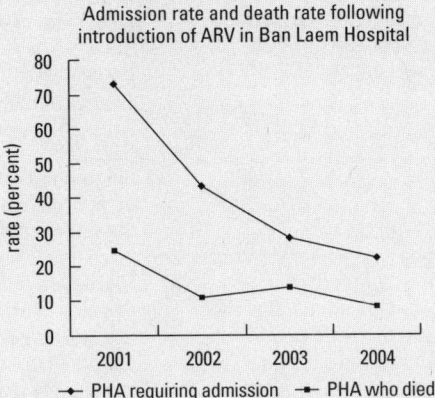

Admission rate and death rate following introduction of ARV in Ban Laem Hospital

*Source:* Wilson and Ford 2004, with help from Chatchai Lalong of Ban Laem Hospital, who provided statistics.

### *Reduces Infectiousness*

Current discussions about the benefits of providing ART to populations in resource-poor countries focus on the ability of ART to reduce the quantity of virus in bodily fluids and therefore to reduce the risk of transmission (Vernazza and others 1999). On the basis of the observed reduction in viral load in blood plasma, experts have predicted that the infectiousness of an HIV-infected person on ART would be reduced by a factor of somewhere between two and eight. That is, the probability of transmission on a single sexual encounter would be reduced to somewhere between 12.5 and 50 percent of its normal value (Over and others 2004). However, evidence on the links between reduced viral load in the plasma and reduced transmission is mixed. Indeed, some recent studies have shown that active virus can be isolated from the genital tract even when there seems to be ade-

**Table 3.8**  Possible Effects of ART on HIV transmission

| Type of effect | | Direction of effect | |
|---|---|---|---|
| | | **Beneficial** *(slows transmission)* | **Adverse** *(speeds up transmission)* |
| Behavioral | | *Reduced infectiousness:* ART may lower viral loads and may therefore lower the risk of transmission per sexual contact. | *Selection for resistance:* Imperfect adherence to ART selects for resistant strains of the virus, which can then be transmitted. *Longer duration of infectivity:* Greater longevity of HIV-infected people taking ART has the unintended negative consequence of increasing the period in which the patient can transmit the virus. |
| Biological | | *Encouragement of prevention, especially diagnostic testing:* ART may increase the uptake rates of prevention activities, particularly voluntary counseling and testing. | *Increased risk behavior:* People receiving ART and HIV-positive and HIV-negative people in the surrounding community may engage in more risky behaviors than they would if ART were unavailable. |

*Source:* Over and others 2004.

quate control of the virus in the blood plasma (Taylor and others 1999; Zhang and others 1998). Several studies have described the concentration of various ART drugs in semen samples. Those studies indicate considerable variation in individual drug levels in semen and no constant relationship between the blood and semen levels.

ART-induced reductions in infectivity depend importantly on how early in the course of the illness PHAs begin therapy. Recent evidence suggests that transmission occurs disproportionately during the first weeks following infection, when most HIV-infected people are unaware of their serostatus (Pilcher and others 2001). However, ART will likely be initiated during the latter stages of the disease, as is recommended by the current WHO guidelines on scaling up of antiretroviral (ARV) drug therapy in resource-limited settings (WHO 2004b). The combination of those factors—residual virus in the genital track, potential for early high transmissibility, and late initiation of ART—could conspire to limit the preventive benefits of ART.[9]

### Encourages Prevention

ART may increase incentives to use preventive services. That possibility is often cited as an argument for expanding the availability of ART in resource-poor countries. The argument is that the availability of effective treatment may encourage people to come forward for VCT. Higher VCT uptake rates would mean that more people would receive prevention counseling and that more HIV-positive people would be detected at an earlier stage of the disease. Those rates could also mean that people who are HIV positive and in need of treatment could start on ART earlier, rather than waiting until they are sick enough to have to access the public health system. However, the actual magnitude of this pro-prevention effect will be highly context specific and will depend on factors such as the size of the increase in the uptake, the risk characteristics of people receiving VCT, and the quality of counseling.

Part of the challenge of using ART as prevention is to encourage people with HIV to be tested early in their illness by attending VCT services, to link those services with ART management, and to ensure good adherence. In Thailand, substantial dissociation remains between VCT and ART management, each of which is the responsibility of different departments of the MOPH. Despite the effort to link those activities, the current focus is largely on expanding the coverage of ART by recruiting patients through the public health system rather than by stimulating the demand for VCT and early recruitment into ART. The scenarios developed in chapter 5 model the potential effect on the epidemic of those two alternative recruitment and expansion strategies.

### Selects for Resistance

In the past few years, the accumulation of evidence derived from studies in industrial countries shows that even modest departures from adherence to ART regimens foster the development of drug-resistant strains of HIV. The presence of drug-resistant strains of HIV in individuals limits the available treatment options and can lead to treatment failure. On a population level, the transmission of resistant strains of HIV may reduce the benefits of an ART distribution program.

A study of 417 participants in four HIV-NAT studies, which included both ART-naive and treatment-experienced patients, showed a rate of virological failure (detectable viral load while taking ART) of 7.8 percent per year of ART. In another cohort of 60 patients who had been exposed to dual therapy and had failed to adhere to it, the virological failure rate was 16 percent per year of ART (Duncombe 2004).

### Increases Risk Behavior

Growing evidence shows that increased availability of ART, together with the perception that there is a "cure" for HIV disease, may lead to a relaxation of efforts to avoid risky behavior. Studies of men who have sex with men (MSM) in Europe and the United States point toward increased risky behavior, such as higher incidence of unprotected anal intercourse and multiple sexual partners (Marseille 2003; Stephenson and others 2003; Stolte and others 2001; Suarez and others 2001; Van de Ven, Kippax, and others 1999; Van de Ven, Rawstorne, and others 2002; Ven 2005).

Comparable evidence for heterosexuals and for MSM in developing countries is scarce. In Brazil, however, the Ministry of Health has pointed to decreased condom use in young MSM, which coincides with the introduction of free ART to all Brazilian citizens, as a factor behind the recent rise in HIV incidence (Over and others 2004). Similarly, a study on the demand for an AIDS vaccine in Thailand suggests that measures perceived to reduce the chances of getting AIDS, such as an effective vaccine, would be associated with negative changes in condom use and risk behavior (Suraratdecha and others 2005).

## Detailed Resource Requirements for ART

Costs of ART can be defined in many ways, such as costs to the public sector, to individual patients, and to the society. In evaluating the various policy options for expanding public provision of ART in Thailand, we adopt the perspective of and estimate the costs to the public sector. This section summarizes the various costs associated with providing ART and presents estimated costs of ART in Thailand.[10] Average costs of ART per patient are estimated on the basis of types of treatment regimens (first-line and second-line therapies); modes of service delivery (public, augmented public, and private service delivery); and stages of the disease (asymptomatic and symptomatic HIV).

Specific components included in estimating average costs of ART per patient are as follows:

- ARV drugs, lab tests, and monitoring

- treatment of OIs

- PHA support.

Cost data were obtained from existing studies in Thailand, both published and unpublished, and from informal consultations with local and international experts.

### Costs of ARV Drugs and Monitoring

Since the production of GPO-vir started in 2002, the GPO has been expanding its production capability and is currently producing five different generic ARV drugs in various forms, combinations, and strengths.[11] That rapid expansion of generic drug production by GPO has greatly affected both access and affordability of ART through NAPHA.

Table 3.9 summarizes costs of various regimens currently available and recommended by the MOPH and WHO in their treatment guidelines. The annual costs of ARV drugs vary significantly between first-line and second-line regimens, ranging from B 14,400 (US$360) (using GPO-vir) to B 273,864 (US$6,847) (using expensive protease inhibitors) per patient per year (Duncombe 2004; GPO 2004). The average cost of a first-line ART regimen is estimated at B 19,271 (US$482) per patient per year, using the weighted average of three categories of ART drug regimens under the MOPH treatment guideline.[12] The average cost of a second-line regimen is estimated around B 270,000 (about US$6,700) per patient, costing nearly 14 times more than the average cost of a first-line regime.

In addition to the cost of ARV drugs, significant costs are associated with providing and monitoring ART treatment. The costs of outpatient and inpatient services are not negligible as use of medical services increases at the time of initiating ART treatment. A recent study[13] evaluating medical resource use for ART, conducted jointly by WHO-Thailand and the Center for Health Economics at Chulalongkorn University in Bangkok, estimated that the average cost of hospital

**Table 3.9**  Costs of ARV Drugs Per Patient by Types of Regimens in Thailand, 2004

| ARV drugs | Monthly cost | | Annual cost | |
|---|---|---|---|---|
| | B | US$ | B | US$ |
| *First-line regimens (MOPH guideline)* | | | | |
| (1) Lamivudine + stavudine + nevirapine | 1,200 | 30.00 | 14,400 | 360.00 |
| (2) Stavudine + lamivudine + efavirenz | 2,579 | 64.50 | 30,948 | 773.70 |
| Zidovudine + lamivudine + efavirenz | 3,819 | 95.50 | 45,828 | 1,145.70 |
| Zidovudine + lamivudine + nevirapine[a] | 2,400 | 60.00 | 28,800 | 720.00 |
| (3) Stavudine + lamivudine + IDV/r | 3,500 | 87.50 | 42,000 | 1,050.00 |
| Zidovudine + lamivudine + IDV/r | 4,740 | 118.50 | 56,880 | 1,422.00 |
| **Average cost** | 1,606 | 40.10 | 19,271 | 481.80 |
| *Second-line regimens (WHO guideline)* | | | | |
| Abacavir + didanosine+ Lopinavir/ritonavir | 22,822 | 570.60 | 273,864 | 6,846.60 |
| Abacavir + didanosine + saquinavir/ritonavir | 22,094 | 552.40 | 265,128 | 6,628.20 |
| **Average cost** | 22,458 | 561.50 | 269,496 | 6,737.40 |

*Source:* Bureau of AIDS, Tuberculosis, and Sexually Transmitted Infection, MOPH, 2004; Duncombe 2004; and GPO 2004.
*Note:* Costs of ARV drugs are based on the lowest prices available, either generic or branded drugs, in Thailand, as of September 2004. US$1 = B 40.
a. The GPO is currently in the process of producing a fixed-dose combination of GPO-Z (zidovudine, lamivudine, and nevirapine). The cost of GPO-Z is approximately B 1,400 (US$35) per month.

services (including outpatient and inpatient services, but excluding ARV drugs, lab tests, and OI medications) is about B 7,700 (US$192.50) per patient per year in public hospitals, ranging from B 12,850 (US$321.25) in university teaching hospitals to B 5,340 (US$133.50) in community hospitals (Supakakunti and others 2004).

The cost of a CD4 test by standard flow cytometry varies from B 200 to B 800 (US$5.00 to US$20.00) with the median cost of B 500

(US$12.50), depending on the institution and the volume of testing. The cost of an HIV RNA (viral-load) test is significantly higher, averaging about B 3,500 (US$87.50) per test. A basic safety chemistry panel measuring serum glutamic oxaloacetic transaminase, creatinine, and glucose costs about B 100 (US$25.00) (Duncombe 2004; Gold and others 2005). In addition to the routine monitoring tests, patients incur sets of screening tests (that is, CD4 counts and HIV antibody tests) before initiation of ART. Those initial screening tests cost about B 1,100 (US$27.50) per patient.

### Cost of OI Treatment

Before the introduction of NAPHA, treatment for OIs comprised the bulk of treatment costs in Thailand's national AIDS expenditure. Existing studies on OI treatment from Thailand were reviewed to estimate the average cost of OI treatment per patient. As discussed in an earlier section, more than 20 different infections are associated with severe immune depletion. Even though the costs of OI treatment vary significantly depending on the type of infection and available treatment options, certain types of infections are observed most often among symptomatic HIV patients. Among the most commonly observed OIs in Thailand are CMV, cryptococcal meningitis, PCP, and TB (Ratanasuwan 2004; Supakakunti and others 2004).

The average costs of OI treatments vary across the studies, ranging from US$64 to US$206 (B 2,560 to B 8,240), with the average cost of US$151 (B 6,040) per patient. To normalize the costs of OI treatment across the studies, we have adjusted those costs by assigning the relative weights of the three most commonly observed OIs (cryptococcal meningitis, PCP, and TB) (see tables B.2 and B.3 in appendix B). Relative weights were calculated in accordance with the prevalence of OIs among AIDS patients in Siriraj University Hospital from 2002 to 2004. Table 3.10 summarizes the estimated annual costs of OI treatment per patient in Thailand.

### Cost of PHA Groups

PHA groups have long played a major role in providing the care and support needed for HIV patients in Thailand. Many of the public hospitals under NAPHA work with PHA groups that provide counseling, information, home visits, and other supports to PHAs. One can expect

**Table 3.10** Average Cost of OI Treatment per Non-ART Patient-Year in Thailand
*2002 US$: 1US$ = B 40*

| Source | | TB | PCP | Cryptococcal meningitis | Total cost |
|---|---|---|---|---|---|
| Honda and others 2002 | Average cost | 45.63 | 35.07 | 131.80 | |
| | Weighted | 20.99 | 10.30 | 32.49 | 63.77 |
| Lertiendumrong, Yenjitr, and Tangcharoensathien 2004 | Average cost | 165.21 | 257.19 | 167.19 | |
| | Weighted | 75.99 | 75.50 | 41.21 | 188.46 |
| Prescott 1995[a] | Average cost | 54.00 | 41.40 | 283.85 | |
| Kongsin and others 2004 | Average cost | 158.55 | 72.45 | 453.30 | |
| | Weighted | 72.93 | 21.27 | 111.72 | 205.92 |
| | Weighted | 24.84 | 12.15 | 69.96 | 104.60 |
| World Bank 1999 | Average cost | 120.15 | 47.66 | 499.35 | |
| | Weighted | 55.26 | 13.99 | 123.07 | 192.33 |

*Note:* Relative weights of 46.0 percent, 29.4 percent, and 24.6 percent are assigned to TB, PCP, and cryptococcal meningitis, respectively.
a. Price figures are updated using the 2004 drug prices in Thailand

that continuous care and support from PHA groups will become increasingly important in expanding public provision of ART, specifically by supporting patients in their adherence to ART. Success of community involvement in HIV/AIDS care through PHA groups and community-based organizations has been well documented in Thailand, although very little has been studied about their resource requirements and financial sustainability. With the help of MSF-Thailand, and drawing on its experience with PHA support groups nationwide, we obtained some preliminary estimates of the costs of PHA support to improve adherence. Those estimates suggest that providing PHA support to improve adherence costs B 3,120 (US$78) per patient (see table 3.11). In other words, such support adds some 7 to 8 percent to the total cost of ART per patient per year (Masaki 2004; Masaki and others 2005)

### *Average Cost of ART per Patient*

The annual cost of ART using first-line therapy is estimated at about B 33,700 (US$843) per patient (see table 3.12). The costs of ARV drugs and lab monitoring equal nearly 60 percent of the total ART cost when first-line therapy is used, whereas the share of ARV drugs

**Table 3.11** Annual Cost of PHA Support Groups per 200 PHA Groups, 2004

| | Annual cost | |
|---|---|---|
| Items | Baht | US$ |
| *Management level* | | |
| Capital items (buildings, vehicles, computers, and so forth) | 98,924 | 2,473 |
| Recurrent items (rents, staff salaries, training costs, maintenance fees, utilities, and so forth) | 6,168,996 | 154,225 |
| *PHA group level* | | |
| Capital items (buildings, vehicles, computers, and so forth) | 550 | 14 |
| Recurrent items (rents, allowances for volunteers, training costs, transportation costs, utilities, and so forth) | 166,500 | 4,163 |
| Total | 6,434,970 | 160,874 |
| Total cost per PHA group | 187,943 | 4,699 |
| Total cost per PHA trained | 62,648 | 1,566 |
| Total cost per client supported | 3,132 | 78 |

*Source:* Thai Network for People Living with HIV/AIDS (TNP+), AIDS Access Foundation, and MSF in Thailand 2004.

and lab tests rises to 95 percent of ART costs when patients are on second-line therapy.

To evaluate costs of various policy options, we have estimated the average costs of ART per patient by modes of service delivery (that is, public and augmented public), by types of drug regimens (first-line and second-line), and by stages of disease (asymptomatic and symptomatic HIV). Those costs are summarized in table 3.13.[14]

**Table 3.12** Annual Cost per Patient by Types of Drug Regimens

| | Annual cost per patient | | | |
|---|---|---|---|---|
| | First-line | | Second-line | |
| Cost items | B | US$ | B | US$ |
| (1) ARV drugs | 18,847 | 471.20 | 263,567 | 6,589.20 |
| (2) Lab tests | 1,210 | 30.30 | 1,210 | 30.30 |
| (3) OI treatment | 4,815 | 120.40 | 4,815 | 120.40 |
| (4) Outpatient service | 2,773 | 69.30 | 2,773 | 69.30 |
| (5) Inpatient service | 6,041 | 151.00 | 6,041 | 151.00 |
| (6) ARV drugs and lab tests: (1) + (2) | 20,057 | 501.40 | 264,778 | 6,619.40 |
| (7) Hospital services: (4) + (5) | 8,815 | 220.40 | 8,815 | 220.40 |
| Total ART cost: (3) + (6) + (7) | 33,688 | 842.20 | 278,408 | 6,960.20 |

*Source:* Supakankunti and others 2004.

**Table 3.13**  Average Costs of ART per Patient by Types of Service Providers, 2004
*Baht*

| ART costs | Public | | | | Augmented Public | | | |
|---|---|---|---|---|---|---|---|---|
| | 1st line | | 2nd line | | 1st line | | 2nd line | |
| | *Asymptomatic* | *Symptomatic* | *Asymptomatic* | *Symptomatic* | *Asymptomatic* | *Symptomatic* | *Asymptomatic* | *Symptomatic* |
| ARV drugs | | | | | | | | |
| 1st-line (MOPH) | 19,271 | 19,271 | | | 19,271 | 19,271 | | |
| 2nd-line (WHO) | | | 269,496 | 269,496 | | | 269,496 | 269,496 |
| Monitoring and lab | 7,824 | 8,568 | 978 | 1,722 | 7,824 | 8,568 | 978 | 1,722 |
| OI Treatment (with ART) | 0 | 4,546 | 0 | 4,546 | 0 | 4,546 | 0 | 4,546 |
| Hospital services | 2,400 | 8,374 | 2,400 | 8,374 | 2,400 | 8,374 | 2,400 | 8,374 |
| OPD service | 2,400 | 2,400 | 2,400 | 2,400 | 2,400 | 2,400 | 2,400 | 2,400 |
| IPD service | 0 | 5,974 | 0 | 5,974 | 0 | 5,974 | 0 | 5,974 |
| PHA support group | | | | | 166,500 | 166,500 | 166,500 | 166,500 |
| Total ART cost/ person month | 2,458 | 3,397 | 22,740 | 23,678 | 16,333 | 17,272 | 36,615 | 37,553 |
| Total ART cost/ person year | 29,495 | 40,758 | 272,874 | 284,137 | 195,995 | 207,258 | 439,374 | 450,637 |

*Source:* Supakankunti and others 2004.
*Note:* The presented cost per patient is an average cost of provincial and community hospitals.

**Notes**

1. For example, see the Concerted Action on Seroconversion to AIDS and Death in Europe (CASCADE) study, which involved 13,030 patients, where the progression rate found a median time to AIDS of 11.0 years (95 percent confidence interval, 10.7–11.7) (CASCADE 2000).

2. According to the World Health Organization (WHO) treatment guidelines, a first-line regimen for HIV should consist of two drugs from the nucleoside reverse transcriptase inhibitor group and one from the nonnucleoside reverse transcriptase inhibitor group. The WHO recommends one of the following four triple-drug combinations for a first-line regimen: (a) stavudine + lamivudine + nevirapine, (b) zidovudine + lamivudine + nevirapine, stavudine + lamivudine + efavirenz, or zidovudine + lamivudine + efavirenz. The WHO recommends that patients shift from a first-line regimen to a second-line regimen if treatment failure occurs. To increase the likelihood of treatment success and to minimize the risk of cross-resistance, the second-line regimen will include at least two new drugs, with at least one from a new class. The WHO-recommended second-line regimen (WHO 2003) is as follows: (a) if stavudine or zidovudine fail, change to tenofovir disoproxil fumarate or abacavir; (b) if lamivudine fails, change to didanosine; and (c) if nevirapine or efavirenz fail, change to lopinavir/ritonavir or saquinavir/ritonavir.

3. The MOPH and the Population Council are now carrying out a more rigorous impact evaluation study of adherence under the National Access to Antiretroviral Program for People Living with HIV/AIDS, in the same Chiang Mai region.

4. GPO-vir comprises stavudine + lamivudine + nevirapine and is given in a dosage of one tablet twice daily. The quantity of stavudine is 40 milligrams twice daily if bodyweight exceeds 60 kilograms (GPO-vir S40) and is 30 milligrams twice daily if bodyweight is less than 60 kilograms (GPO-vir S30).

5. The 2NN study is an open-label comparative study to evaluate the antiviral efficacy and safety of using nevirapine and efavirenz or

both drugs combined in combination with stavudine and lamivudine. It was presented at the 10th Conference on Retroviruses and Opportunistic Infections, held in Boston on February 10-14, 2003.

6. David Wilson, MSF, personal communication, Bangkok 2005.

7. Personal communications with Chris Duncombe (Thai Red Cross/HIV-NAT), Julian Gold (Albion Street Clinic), and David Wilson (MSF), Bangkok 2005.

8. This discussion draws heavily from Over and others (2004).

9. Wawer and others (2005) provide data that support the reverse J-shaped pattern of infectivity with high initial infectivity, followed by low infectivity for many years before the onset of AIDS symptoms. They conclude that ART will have little effect on infectivity.

10. This section draws heavily from Masaki (2004).

# CHAPTER 4

# The Effects of Thailand's
# Current AIDS Policy

The evolution of Thailand's AIDS policy and the main features of its current policy for treatment (National Access to Antiretrovirals Program for People Living with AIDS, or NAPHA) are described in chapters 2 and 3. This chapter first presents a framework for analyzing the effect of government policy and then presents projections of the costs and effects of the NAPHA policy in comparison with a baseline projection of what would have happened in the absence of NAPHA. The considerable fiscal burden of the NAPHA policy is projected and compared with the total health budget and the total AIDS budget.

## Framework for AIDS Policy Analysis

Governments implement policies by wielding one or more policy instruments under their control. These instruments can be grouped as follows:

- technical or engineering instruments, such as draining wetlands to combat malaria

- legal instruments, which give citizens both rights and obligations and must be enforced by a judicial system

- voluntary or behavioral instruments, which give people new information or change the prices or other incentives that guide their behavior.

Because the risky sexual and drug-using behaviors that transmit sexually transmitted diseases are private or even clandestine activities, technical and legal instruments have little force to prevent transmission. Government prevention programs have largely relied on behavioral instruments, such as providing information about the danger of HIV infection or subsidizing the prices of condoms. The discovery of a vaccine against AIDS would provide governments with a technical instrument, but inducing people to be vaccinated may require behavioral instruments.

At first glance, treatment with antiretroviral therapy (ART) may seem to be a purely technical instrument to address the damaging consequences of AIDS. However, Thailand's goals of expanding treatment to all HIV-infected residents with CD4 counts less than 200 cells per cubic millimeter and maintaining those people in good health as long as possible are ambitious. Achieving them will require the country to use all available instruments. In launching NAPHA, the government has already used the technical instrument of producing GPO-vir and the legal instrument of authorizing its production. It has mandated that government health facilities offer voluntary counseling and testing (VCT) for HIV infection, CD4 tests for those who are infected, and treatment for the eligible. By offering the treatment at nominal charges, it is also using a price instrument. The exercise of these instruments has resulted in a remarkable scale-up of treatment—from fewer than 3,000 persons living with HIV/AIDS (PHAs) under publicly financed ART in 2001 to more than 50,000 in early 2005. The challenge is to maintain those patients in good health for as long as possible.

### From Policies to Epidemiology to Performance

To estimate the outcome of NAPHA and then the cost-effectiveness of various modifications of it, we must model how the specific changes introduced by this policy influence the behavior of patients and providers. Our approach is to construct a model of the links between government instruments and policy outcomes.

We do this in five steps (figure 4.1):

- *Step 1.* We model the link from the two primary policy instruments, price and availability (or supply), to the distribution of patient demand for care.

- *Step 2.* We project the evolution of prices and availability into the future and compute the projected distribution of demand across treatment options.

- *Step 3.* We apply the expected demand to the population of eligible infected people, as projected by an updated version of the Asian Epidemic Model (AEM), to deduce the future use of ART.

- *Step 4.* We estimate the direct and indirect health benefits of ART use.

- *Step 5.* We apply the unit costs from chapter 3 to estimate the financial burden of the NAPHA policy.

In this chapter, these five steps are applied to the NAPHA policy and to the baseline as a comparator. In chapter 5, using the same model, we apply steps 2 through 5 to three modified versions of the NAPHA policy. We then compare the stream of future health benefits with the stream of future costs for NAPHA and for three alternatives and estimate the cost-effectiveness of each version of the NAPHA policy.

**Figure 4.1** From Polices to Epidemiology to Performance

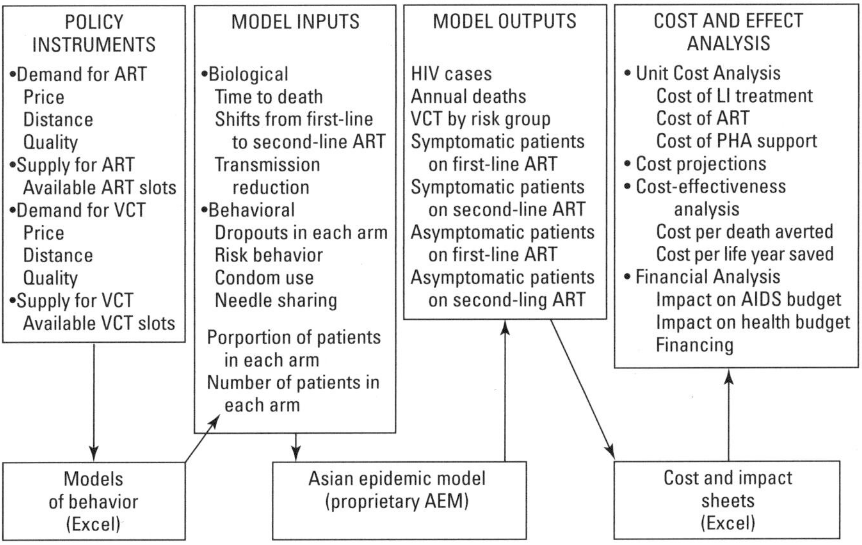

*Source:* Authors.
*Note:* OI = opportunistic infection.

## Modeling the Effects of Policy Instruments

The demand for a health service is typically modeled by relating the quantity demanded to the price the patient must pay for the service, the distance he or she must travel, the quality of the care, and other relevant attributes (Akin, Guilkey, and Denton 1995; Akin and others 1998; Christianson 1976; Cissé 2004; Gertler and van der Gaag 1990; Levy and Germain 1994; Litvack and Bodart 1993; Mwabu, Ainsworth, and Nyamete 1993; Mwabu and Mwangi 1986).[1] Because a sick person's knowledge of the quality and effectiveness of a health service can also influence demand, the effect of information about quality should be modeled as well. Figure 4.2 illustrates the assumption that these four variables and others affect a symptomatic AIDS patient's decision about whether to seek treatment and which of three treatment options to choose.

It is unfortunately quite possible for some patients to choose not to seek treatment for an illness, even if they have good information. The option of no treatment is especially likely among poor people in a poor country, for whom only a few kilometers or the price of food at a health facility can be insuperable obstacles. Patients residing in urban centers usually have a choice of alternative providers and treatment options, referred to in the model as *public treatment* or *private treatment*. Typically the distinguishing features of private facilities are higher prices and greater confidentiality. Patients in rural areas may have available only one facility in each class, and sometimes the closest private facility will be quite far away. A third option, *augmented public treatment*, consists of standard public treatment with the addition of a government-subsidized nongovernmental organization (NGO) to help patients adhere to the prescribed behaviors and medications.

**Figure 4.2**  Choice of Treatment Mode among Symptomatic HIV-Positive Adults

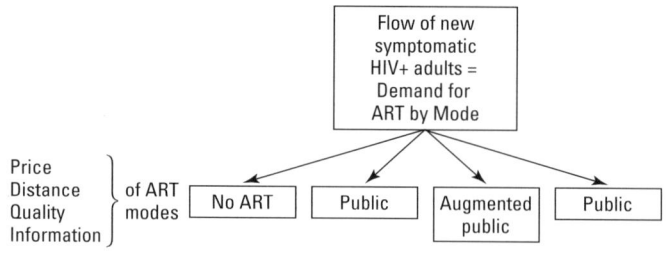

*Source:* Authors.

This third option has existed in Thailand for more than a decade because of the initiative of international NGOs such as Médecins sans Frontières (MSF). The concept of the grant-subsidized support group, typically consisting of persons living with HIV/AIDS (PHAs), has recently received endorsement from the government and financial support from the Global Fund to Fight AIDS, Tuberculosis, and Malaria. The number of such groups is thus expanding.

To move from the conceptual model of figure 4.2 to a simulation model capable of plausibly describing and predicting real-world behavior, we must choose a functional representation of the impact of price, availability, and other variables on the patient's choice of treatment mode. To avoid the complexity of feedback from the epidemiological model to the demand model, we will assume that mode characteristics affect the proportion of patients choosing each mode without regard to the number of such patients.[2] Furthermore, we seek a functional form that guarantees that under any combination of mode characteristics the proportions of patients choosing the four treatment modes adds to unity (to 1.0). The functional form most frequently adopted in the literature is that of the multinomial logit, which has a respected history of modeling consumers' choices among multiple alternatives partly because it has these two desirable characteristics.[3] In our application, the demand for public ART using this functional form is written as follows:

$$q\_pub\_art = \frac{e^{(\alpha\_pub + \beta \cdot LN(Ppub\_art) + \gamma \cdot LN(Dpub\_art))}}{\sum_e (\alpha\_x\_art + \beta \cdot LN(Px\_art) + \gamma \cdot LN(Dx\_art))}$$

$$x = \{ pub, apub, priv, no\}$$

where
LN denotes the natural logarithm
$e$ denotes the base of the natural logarithms
$q\_pub\_art$ = the proportion of patients choosing public ART
$Px\_art$ = the price paid by patients for delivery mode $x$, defined as one of the following:
$pub$ = public mode of ART delivery
$apub$ = augmented public mode of ART delivery
$priv$ = private mode of ART delivery
$no$ = treatment for opportunistic infections without ART

Similarly:

> $Dx\_art$ = the average distance from patients to delivery mode $x$, as defined above
>
> $\alpha x\_art$ = a constant that captures all other features of mode $x$ that influence the patient's choice, such as quality and information
>
> $\beta$ = the elasticity of patients' demand to price
>
> $\gamma$ = the elasticity of patients' demand to distance.

The demand functions for the other three modes look the same except that the mode designation *pub* in the dependent variable and in the numerator is replaced by the appropriate mode designation.[4]

The variables *Ppub_art*, *Dpub_art*, *Papub_art*, *Dapub_art*, *Pno_art*, and *Dno_art* are all policy instruments that the government can manipulate to affect patient mode choice. Hence, our alternative scenarios consist of alternative projections of these variables. To predict the pattern over time of the share of patients across modes, one must choose values of the $\beta$ and $\gamma$ parameters and of the four values for $\alpha\_x$. We have calibrated these parameters for two groups of patients: the symptomatic and the asymptomatic. Table 4.1 gives the two elasticities and four intercept values for each patient category.

The elasticity parameters can be interpreted as the percentage change in the odds ratio between two mode choices in response to a 1 percent change in the ratio of their prices or distances.[5] Therefore, the elasticity of –0.5 of symptomatic people to the price of ART means that the odds of a person choosing any of the modes over another falls by 0.5 percent for every 1 percent increase in the price ratio between the modes.[6] Because sick people have difficulty travel-

**Table 4.1** Calibrated Values of the Parameters That Characterize Patient Choice of Treatment Mode in Thailand

| Parameter | Patient category | |
| --- | --- | --- |
| | *Symptomatic* | *Asymptomatic* |
| Price elasticities | –0.50 | –1.00 |
| Distance elasticities | –1.50 | –0.50 |
| *Intercepts* | | |
| Public ART | 7.08 | 4.42 |
| Augmented public ART | 8.14 | 3.52 |
| Private ART | 10.15 | 4.49 |
| No ART | 1.00 | 1.00 |

*Source:* Authors' calibration of Thai historical aggregated data for 2001–3.

ing, we assume that they will be quite responsive to distance, with a calibrated elasticity of –1.5. The intercept parameters are normalized at a value of 1 for no ART. The ratios of the other intercepts to the "no ART" intercept reflect the perceived desirability or subjective quality of care in the patients' eyes. Given the effectiveness of ART in relieving symptoms and prolonging life, it is not surprising that the intercept parameters for all three treatment options are much larger than for the "no ART" option. Among the three treatment options, private care seems to rank highest, perhaps because of the greater confidentiality as well as the personalized service. Augmented public is next largest while pure public is somewhat smaller, perhaps reflecting a perception that augmentation by an NGO improves the effectiveness of care.

Figure 4.2 depicts our conceptual model of the decision to seek treatment made by a person who is suffering symptoms of AIDS (symptomatic HIV-positive) and visits health care facilities to seek alleviation of that suffering. Most patients who seek treatment in Thailand fall in this category and have advanced AIDS disease with CD4 counts of 50 cells per cubic millimeter or below. However, current medical opinion holds that the optimal time to begin ART is significantly earlier, when the patient's CD4 count has dropped from its normal level of between 600 and 1,000 to a level of 200 cells per cubic millimeters. Most such patients are still symptom-free and would be unaware of the benefit they could obtain from ART, unless they had taken a test for HIV infection. The path to treatment for these asymptomatic patients thus begins with the demand for VCT.

Figure 4.3 illustrates our conceptual model of this route into treatment. The individual must first decide to seek out the VCT service, a decision that depends on the characteristics of those services and on the patient's information about them. Once the individual learns that he or she is HIV positive, a count of the density of CD4 cells in his or her blood determines whether treatment should be started. Asymptomatic patients who demand care have passed through these two filters.

We model the first filter (VCT) using a demand curve like that for ART but simplified to include only two options: "seek VCT" and "do not seek VCT." Again, the policy instruments available to government include a price and a distance, the price of VCT and the average distance to it. But in addition to these two instruments, which act directly on the demand for VCT, we posit that patients demand more VCT if

**Figure 4.3** Demand for Voluntary Counseling and Testing and Choice of Treatment Mode among Asymptomatic HIV-Positive Adults

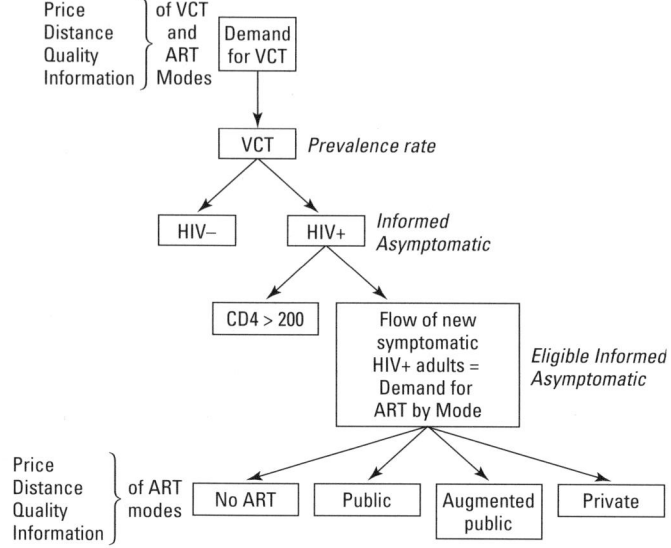

*Source:* Authors.

the price of and the distance to public ART are lower. This assumption captures the frequently suggested hypothesis that people are more willing to learn their HIV status if they know that treatment is available to those who test positive.[7] Accordingly, in our model, policies followed by the government to encourage ART also encourage VCT.

The demand for VCT depends not only on characteristics of its supply but also on characteristics of prospective candidates. People who believe that they have been exposed to HIV through risky behavior have a greater incentive to seek information about their serostatus, especially when ART is available. The reverse is true among low-risk people, who may be hard to convince to seek VCT. To capture the difference between these two populations of consumers, we specify and calibrate separate demand curves for high-risk and low-risk groups.

The calibrated values of the parameters of the VCT demand function are given in table 4.2. The selected values of these parameters reflect our belief that the high-risk group is highly responsive to the availability of ART—more so than the low-risk group, which does not perceive itself to be in danger. In contrast, the low-risk group is highly responsive to the price of VCT but less likely to consider the price of

**Table 4.2** Calibrated Values of the Parameters That Characterize Patient Choice of VCT

| | Risk group | |
| --- | --- | --- |
| **Parameters** | **Low risk** | **High risk** |
| *Price elasticities* | | |
| Price elasticity of VCT | −1.5 | −0.2 |
| Price elasticity of ART | −0.4 | −0.6 |
| *Distance elasticities* | | |
| Distance elasticity of VCT | −1.5 | −0.2 |
| Distance elasticity of ART | −0.4 | −0.6 |
| Intercepts | −12.2 | −2.2 |

*Source:* Authors' calibration of Thai historical aggregated data for 2001–3.

ART in making the decision. For lack of information, we assume the same elasticities for both prices and distances. The values of the intercepts reflect our belief that the high-risk group is much more likely to be tested than the low-risk group.

Once VCT candidates receive their results, they learn whether they are HIV positive or negative. Those who are positive learn whether they have CD4 counts lower than 200 cells per cubic millimeter and thus are eligible for ART. The demand function for these asymptomatic people is given by the parameters in the second data column of table 4.1.

When the supply of ART is less than the demand for it, shortages and rationing will result. Market-clearing mechanisms in such circumstances might include price increases (legal and illegal), longer queuing times, or quality reductions. In the case of acute illness episodes of other diseases—such as food poisoning, acute upper respiratory infections, or malaria—demand is brief, lasting only a few days per episode. Supply must occur simultaneously with demand for an equally brief period. For such diseases, both supply and demand can be modeled as flows of episodes per year. However, once a person starts ART, that person must—with only minor exceptions—remain on ART for the rest of his or her life. In this respect, ART resembles kidney dialysis for those with kidney failure and insulin therapy for diabetics. For all these diseases, the flow of new demand for care in a given year is additional to the stock of demand remaining in the system from previous years. To satisfy all this demand, the stock of available ART treatment slots must equal or exceed the stock of patients demanding ART.

The models we have presented for the demand for ART and for the demand for VCT are models of flows. The demand for VCT is modeled as a proportion of all HIV-negative adults.[8] The demand for ART by asymptomatic people is modeled as a proportion of those who know that they are HIV positive and learn in a given year that they have a CD4 count less than 200 cells per cubic millimeter and are thus eligible for ART. The demand for ART by symptomatic people is modeled as a proportion of those whose CD4 counts fall for the first time below a critical level of 50 cells per cubic millimeter, a level that we assume is on average associated with the onset of AIDS symptoms. Because some people develop symptoms that lead to AIDS treatment before their CD4 counts drop this low, this assumption underestimates the total demand by symptomatic patients and therefore leads to underestimates of government expenditure.

Our assumption about the supply of VCT services is simply that a sufficient flow will be available in unlimited quantities to meet demand at a fixed unit cost. For ART, however, we must take into account that supply is a stock of treatment slots and demand for those slots is expressed by a stock of eligible patients, including some who have been on ART for some time and others who are newly eligible or have been eligible for a while but unable to find a treatment slot. Figure 4.4 illustrates how we compute the actual amount of ART delivered by comparing the stocks of ART supply and ART demand.

The procedure for allocating treatment slots is guided by a policy rule that derives from the conventional medical rule to tend first to those in direst need. We assume that patients who were under treatment the previous year have first priority for treatment slots unless they are lost to follow-up or die. Available treatment slots are then assigned in order of priority so that a specified percentage ($X$) of slots go to the new flow of demand by symptomatic patients and the remaining percentage of slots are available to the new flow of demand from eligible asymptomatic patients. If the government were able to reassign available treatment slots instantly around the country to meet year-to-year fluctuations of demand by newly symptomatic patients, then $X$ might be set to 100 percent. In this case, the model would describe a situation in which all demand by symptomatic patients anywhere in the country would be satisfied before the first asymptomatic patient is treated anywhere by the public sector. However, we set $X$ to 90 percent to capture the difficulty of achieving such instantaneous reassignment or an inten-

**Figure 4.4** Supply and Demand for ART by Treatment Mode

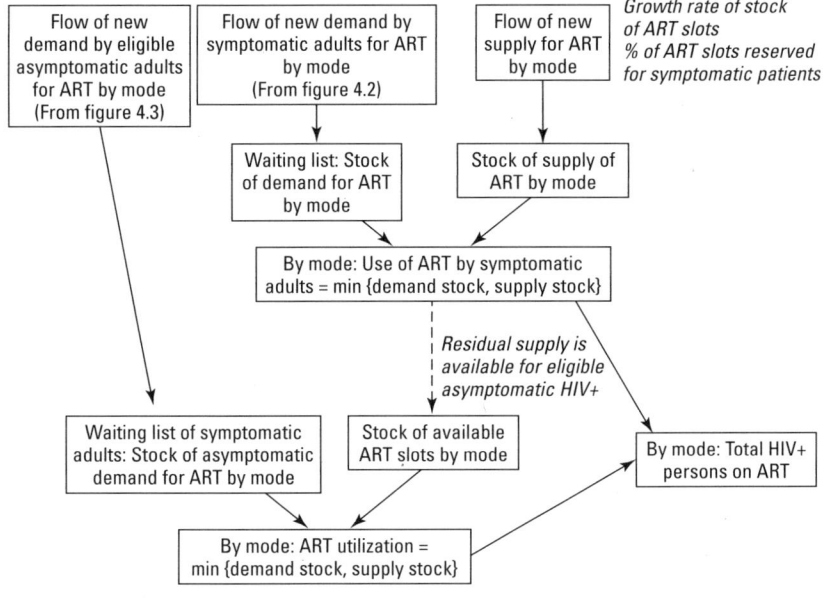

*Source:* Authors.

tional government policy of treating some people when their CD4 counts are above 100 cells per cubic millimeter. This assumption that 90 percent of slots go first to symptomatic patients is maintained across all the simulated policy scenarios both here and in chapter 5.

In summary, the policy part of our model takes as inputs the policy instruments listed in table 4.3 and provides as outputs to the epidemiological model the variables listed in table 4.4. The input variables subject to government control are primarily prices and distances to testing and treatment facilities. The output variables are the proportions of various population groups that seek VCT or ART in a given year and the availability of ART treatment slots for all the accumulated people demanding care.

The assumptions about the functional form of the demand equations and the calibrated values of the elasticities and other demand parameters are based on the limited data available. In the future, it may be possible to collect microeconomic data on households that are actually making the choices modeled here. Then these data could be used to estimate the values of these demand parameters and to choose the best-fitting functional forms for the demand functions. Since such data are

**Table 4.3**  Major Policy Inputs to the Policy Model That Generate Alternative Scenarios: 18 Projected Variables

| | HIV-positive population | | HIV-negative population (CD4 < 200 cells/mm³) | |
|---|---|---|---|---|
| | **Low risk** | **High risk** | **Informed asymptomatic** | **Symptomatic** |
| Demand for VCT | Price and distance to VCT (2 variables) | Price and distance to VCT (same 2 variables) | n.a. | n.a. |
| Demand for ART | n.a. | n.a. | Price and distance to ART by treatment mode (2 variables) | Price and distance to ART by treatment mode (same 2 variables) |
| Supply of VCT | Unlimited | Unlimited | n.a. | n.a. |
| Supply of ART | n.a. | n.a. | Growth rate of facilities (average slots per facility), by treatment mode | Growth rate of facilities (average slots per facility), by treatment mode |

*Source:* Authors.
*Note:* n.a. = not applicable.

not currently available, we impose more theoretical structure on the problem, to provide plausible projections of the alternative scenarios.

We model government policy options as affecting the future performance of ART delivery through government-mandated changes in the prices of public and augmented public ART, in the provision of public ART, and in the provision and financing of augmented public ART. These mandated changes directly affect demand through the price and distance variables, as described above. They also affect supply (for example, the total available treatment slots). The policy workbook part of our model captures these processes by generating a time series of input values for the epidemiological model. The 18 time series variables generated are shown in table 4.4.

## An Overview of the AEM

### The Model

The AEM is a difference equation model that projects the dynamic patterns of HIV epidemics in Asian settings. Developed by Brown and Peerapatanapokin of the East-West Center, in collaboration with the

**Table 4.4**  Outputs from the Policy Model That Drive the AEM for Each Scenario: 18 Projected Variables

| | HIV-positive population | | HIV-negative population (CD4 < 200 cells/mm³) | |
|---|---|---|---|---|
| | Low risk | High risk | Informed asymptomatic | Symptomatic |
| Demand for VCT | Proportion demanding VCT (1 variable) | Proportion demanding VCT (1 variable) | n.a. | n.a. |
| Demand for ART | n.a. | n.a. | Proportion demanding each mode (4 variables) | Proportion demanding each mode (4 variables) |
| Supply of VCT | Unlimited | Unlimited | n.a. | n.a. |
| Supply of ART | n.a. | n.a. | Minimum slots for each treatment mode (4 variables) | Maximum slots for each treatment mode (4 variables) |

*Source:* Authors' construction.
*Note:* n.a. = not applicable.

Thai Working Group on HIV/AIDS Projection and the Ministry of Public Health (MOPH), the model is sufficiently disaggregated to benefit from available data on risk behavior and HIV prevalence in all the important risk groups in the Thai population (Brown and Peerapatanapokin 2004b; Thai Working Group on HIV/AIDS Projection 2001). Before the addition of modules to capture ART, versions of the AEM were presented to and reviewed by attendees at several international conferences and at meetings of the Joint United Nations Programme on HIV/AIDS (UNAIDS) Reference Group on Epidemiology. The biological parameters of the model have been calibrated so that the model's projected prevalence rates match observed rates by risk group.[9] Such detailed fitting is rare among models of HIV epidemics, partly because most countries outside Thailand have too few data to permit such comparisons.

The model has three major transmission modules: heterosexual contact, needle sharing, and homosexual male-to-male contact. These components are subdivided into eight populations:

• male clients of sex workers

• male nonclients of sex workers

• male injecting drug users (IDUs) with high needle sharing

- male IDUs with low needle sharing

- men who have sex with men

- female direct sex workers

- female indirect sex workers

- female nonsex workers (that is, the general female population).

Interactions of these subpopulations are illustrated in figure 4.5.

Each of these subpopulations is further divided into those who are infected (HIV positive) and those who are susceptible to infection (HIV negative). The AEM calculates HIV infection in the seronegative members of each risk group as driven by that group's risky contacts with the other groups and the HIV seroprevalence in each of those other groups. The model also makes assumptions about transitions from one risk group to another.[10] These assumptions allow the model to capture the common observation that individuals are not permanently identifiable as members of a specific risk group but change their behavior over their life cycles. Heterosexual men are likely to visit sex workers more frequently when they are single than when they are married; many female sex workers practice their trade for only a few years before retiring to get married; men who have sex with men—and, indeed, all adults—have fewer partners when they get older (Brown and Peerapatanapokin 2004b; Guest, du Guerny, and Hsu 2003).

**Figure 4.5**  Stylized Structure of the AEM: Transmission

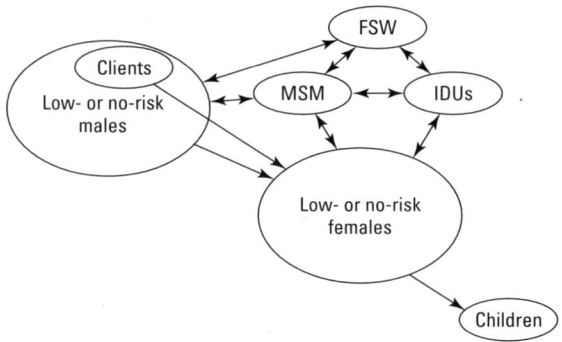

*Source:* Brown 2004.
*Note:* FSW = female sex workers.
MSM = men who have sex with men.

New infections in any given group are hence a function of eight quantitative factors, all but one of which changes over time. For example, consider the equation for the rate of new infections among the uninfected male clients of female sex workers. This infection rate is affected by numerous factors:[11]

- the prevalence of HIV among sex workers

- the fraction of sex acts that are not protected by condoms

- the frequency of contact (that is, the frequency of the client's willingness to pay for sex with a sex worker)

- the proportion of clients who are circumcised

- the reduction in the probability of infection attributable to circumcision

- the proportion of clients who have a classic sexually transmitted infection (STI) such as syphilis or gonorrhea

- the degree to which such an STI amplifies transmission probability.

The one constant parameter in the model, the biological rate of transmission between an infected and an uninfected person in the two contact groups, is calibrated so that the projected incidence, prevalence, and behavioral patterns match the observed historical time paths for these variables.

Among the most important behavioral input variables included in the model are

- sizes of key populations over time—for example, total population, number of 15-year-olds in each year, IDUs, men who have sex with men, and direct and indirect sex workers

- frequency of risk behaviors, including sex with various partner types, sharing of needles, and so on

- levels of protective behaviors—for example, use of condoms among different risk groups, use of clean needles, and percentage of men who are circumcised (Thai Working Group on HIV/AIDS Projection 2001).

*Asian Epidemic Model with ART*
Until 2002, the number of patients on ART in Thailand was too small to have a significant effect on the prevalence rate of HIV infection or

on the rate of new infections (incidence). As a result of the Thai government's decision to adopt the NAPHA policy, both the numbers of people receiving treatment and the presumed effectiveness of treatment have dramatically improved. Accordingly, it is no longer possible to make reasonable projections about the course of the epidemic without including the effects of ART. The authors of the AEM joined the report team to model as accurately as possible the potential effects of ART policy on ART use and the effects of ART implementation on the course of the epidemic. This collaboration came about for two reasons:

• to update the AEM to current and future epidemiological realities

• to respond to the Thai government's request to model the costs and effects of their new treatment policies and its possible variants.

It has led to the development of a new "policy workbook" model to capture the effect of policy on ART use and to a revised version of the AEM that integrates into the model the complexities of the Thai system for providing ART.

The ART components of the revised AEM build on earlier work to integrate ART into a simpler differential equation model of the AIDS epidemic in India (Over and others 2004). However, the ART components of the AEM differ from that earlier work in important ways that reflect Thailand's greater experience with public sector ART provision, its ability to afford a more generous ART treatment protocol, recognition of the challenges that all countries confront in recruiting patients before their disease advances to the point that they are difficult to help, and the more sophisticated modeling foundation of the AEM.

Figure 4.6 uses the ART component of the model for male clients of sex workers as an example of how ART processes are appended to the epidemiological superstructure of the AEM. The left side of the figure is a simple representation of the epidemiological part of the model for clients. The first new feature introduced to the model because of ART is the possibility that the client will be infected with a strain of HIV that is resistant to ART. Such strains did not exist at significant levels in Thailand until the advent of the new, ambitious treatment policy. One reason for adding ART to the AEM is to project the effect of various ART policies on the spread of such resistant strains. In the present implementation of the AEM, we assume for simplicity that people

**Figure 4.6** Client Compartment of the AEM with ART

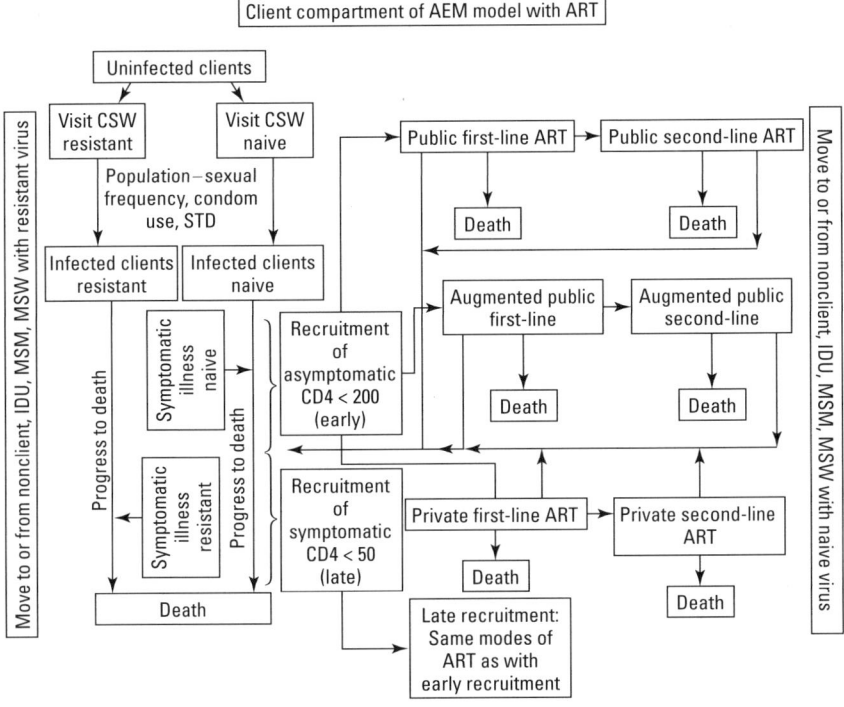

Source: Authors.
Note: MSM = men who have sex with men, MSW = male sex workers, CSW = commercial sex workers.

infected with a resistant strain do not benefit from ART and therefore do not use it. As Thailand continues to gather information on the prevalence of resistant strains and as the public sector develops and widely implements therapeutic protocols for such patients, the AEM can be modified to include those additional complexities.

The numerically more important branch on the right side of figure 4.6 is infection with a naive (or "wild" or "susceptible") strain of HIV. The progression of disease in these patients is modeled as an inexorable process according to the natural history assumptions detailed in chapter 3, unless it is interrupted by treatment. The HIV-infected person has two opportunities to be recruited for treatment. If the person seeks VCT and learns that he (or in other compartments of the model, she) is infected and has a CD4 count below 200 cells per cubic millimeter, that person might choose to seek treatment relatively early during the illness (from two to six years after infection). The AEM captures here the outcome of the choice process that is modeled in the policy workbook model and described above.

Once the person is recruited into ART and selects one of the three treatment modes, he or she follows the progression to treatment failure or to dropping out of treatment that is characteristic of that treatment mode and recruitment time. The figure displays the possibilities of remaining in first-line therapy, dropping out of it, moving on to second-line therapy, or dying. From second-line therapy, the figure displays the possibilities of remaining in therapy, dropping out, or dying. Those progression probabilities are modeled as described in chapter 3 and are based on all available data and on the expert opinions of the clinicians on the report team and among the background paper authors.

If the person does not learn his or her HIV status or, despite learning that he or she is positive and eligible, chooses not to seek early treatment, the person can again be recruited for treatment when he or she becomes symptomatic at CD4 counts below 50 cells per cubic millimeter. The decision to seek treatment at this late stage is again modeled in the policy workbook. The outcome of individual decisions is captured here in the AEM by the box labeled "late recruitment." The structure of treatment options available to patients at late recruitment is identical to those available at early recruitment.[12] However, as described above, progression to treatment failure and disease is more rapid for the average patient than it would have been if he or she had begun treatment with a more intact immune system. Also, the public health care system is presumed to give priority to symptomatic patients if it is ever short of treatment slots. We assume that only 10 percent of treatment slots are reserved for early treatment regardless of the size of the asymptomatic waiting list.[13]

### Measuring the Performance of ART Policy

The objective of ART policy is to improve the health of patients, allowing them to live longer, healthier lives. But ART policy has other effects—some beneficial to the patient and society and some potentially harmful. A full economic analysis of ART would attach a monetary value to all of its effects, whether beneficial or harmful, to compute the net present value of the policy. Such an aggregated perspective is especially useful for comparing the social rate of return on investments in treating AIDS patients with the return on investments in other sectors. The disadvantage of adopting the full economic approach lies in the fact that unit values for healthy life-years, years of orphanhood, and other effects of the ART policy are hard to establish or defend. Analysis based on controversial unit values is itself controversial, and this controversy may distract from points that can be made without adopting these monetary values. So in this analysis we have chosen to keep track of as many effects of ART as possible, without attempting to aggregate them across categories. Our approach fits within the framework of cost-effectiveness analysis rather than cost-benefit analysis.

*Effects*

Before the advent of ART in developing countries, the best indicator of the spread of HIV infection was the prevalence of infection in the population. Although economists and epidemiologists have complained that the best measure of the effectiveness of AIDS prevention policy would be the change in the incidence rate (that is, the rate of new infections), data on the incidence of HIV is so rare that prevalence was used in its place (World Bank 1999). Typically, a decrease in the prevalence rate was interpreted to mean that the incidence rate must be smaller than the rate of death of HIV-infected people. This was the pattern observed in Thailand in the 1990s (World Bank 2000). In the absence of ART, an increase in prevalence could be interpreted to mean only that the incidence was higher than the death rate. This situation could occur in a country such as South Africa, where infection spread rapidly before the death rate caught up, or in a country with a longer history of widespread infection because incidence continues to increase. In either case, in the absence of effective AIDS treatment, rising prevalence would always be bad news.

The presence of ART has reversed the interpretation that must be placed on increasing prevalence levels. By keeping infected people alive longer, ART maintains a prevalence rate even if incidence falls to zero. With a small incidence rate and an effective ART program, prevalence will continue to rise. Prevalence retains its value as an index of the current and potential future burden of the epidemic on the country's health care system, but it loses its value as an indicator of the effectiveness of an HIV prevention policy.

The number of deaths is an index of the effectiveness of an ART program that is particularly useful in the short run. In the years immediately following the introduction of ART access, the number of annual deaths falls almost one for one with the number of treatment slots made available. However, deaths are not a valid index of the continuing benefits of an ART program over the long run. Because everyone dies eventually, comparing a future without ART to one with ART shows the effect of ART to be fewer deaths in the near future and then even more deaths in the more distant future. This effect occurs because the cohort of people placed on ART at the beginning of the program begin to die, which adds their deaths to those of the HIV-negative people whose dates of death are not affected by the ART program. It will appear that the ART program is causing deaths a decade after its introduction, when it is actually having the beneficial effect of shifting the deaths forward in time. Hence, the number of deaths averted, like HIV prevalence, is an unappealing measure of the effectiveness of an AIDS treatment policy.

Because the objective of ART policy is to lengthen and improve the lives of the recipients, a natural measure of the effectiveness of a policy is the number of life-years it adds to the population. With a microsimulation model, such a measure is easy to implement by simply keeping track of the number of life-years lived by each individual and comparing the aggregate of these life-years between two runs of the model: one with ART and one without it. Because the AEM is a difference equation model, in which individuals are subsumed into groups, it is not possible to directly measure the life-years saved. However the model does provide a count of the number of people beginning ART at each of the two recruitment points: early and late. Figure 3.4 in chapter 3 presented a calculation of the estimated number of additional life-years that accrue to each individual who begins treatment, sorted by whether that treatment is early or late. We measure the effectiveness of an ART policy option by multiplying this estimate of per patient life-year benefit by the number of patients initiating each type of treatment in that year. This method gives a stream of annual benefits that continues over time as long as treatment continues.

Another potential benefit of ART is that children are not orphaned until they are older and farther along in their transition to independence. That this benefit is potentially important, not only for the psychological well-being of the children directly concerned but also for national economic growth, has been demonstrated in a recent series of papers by Bell, Devarajan, and Gersback (2004). However, the AEM is not a full demographic model and therefore does not capture fertility in a realistic way. The report team has not attempted to estimate the years of orphanhood that would be saved by ART treatment.[14]

Chapter 3 described the possible effects of ART on preventing new HIV infections. Through the biological channel, ART might either slow transmission (by reducing the viral load in bodily fluids) or accelerate it (through greater or longer sexual activity of the infected person). Through the behavioral channel, ART could also have either beneficial effects (by encouraging the demand for VCT) or negative effects (if people relax their efforts to prevent infection in response to better availability of high-quality treatment). Furthermore, the degree of adherence practiced by the average ART patient also affects the spread of resistant strains of the virus—a potentially dangerous negative spillover effect of treatment on others. The index of all of these effects is the rate of new HIV infections or the HIV incidence rate.

In principle, it is desirable to measure the effects of ART policy on the distribution of the burden of HIV/AIDS by income category. It is often asserted (with little empirical support) that the Thai HIV epidemic mainly affects the poor. If this assertion is true, a generous ART subsidy might be equity enhancing, helping the poor more than the rich. However, the AEM does not distinguish groups of people by socioeconomic status. Accordingly, it affords little opportunity for analyzing the equity effects of alternative ART policies. However, chapter 5 considers some equity implications of NAPHA based on population averages.

In comparing alternative AIDS policies, our analytical techniques must recognize that the effects of current policies persist for a long time. When the Thai government buys vehicles, it can hope that they last five years. Roads last 5 or 10 years, and buildings last 15 or more years. However, the consequences of AIDS treatment policy will last even longer, as cohorts of people remain alive rather than dying, infect or don't infect others, and continue to consume medical care for as long as three decades after beginning treatment. Therefore, it is essential to adopt a long-term perspective in measuring the effects of alternative polices. To consistently compare scenarios in which the benefits and costs occur at different points in time, this report applies standard discounting formulas to future streams of benefits and costs to convert them to their present values (World Bank 1993).[15]

*Costs*

Cost analysis of health programs typically distinguishes between fixed costs and variable costs. The fixed costs are occasioned by the establishment of a health program, while the variable costs are typically unit costs multiplied by the number of units of output. In this simple cost model, the fixed costs are spread over all the units of output, leading to the phenomenon of increasing *economies of scale:* the more units of output produced, the lower the cost per unit of output. When programs are added to existing programs, costs are typically saved because some of the fixed and variable costs of the new program can be avoided by using existing facilities and resources. Economies of this sort are called *economies of scope.* When a program is expanded beyond its most efficient scale or extra programs added to existing ones get in the way of one another, diseconomies of scale or of scope can also appear. The question is whether the Thai ART program will experience economies of scale or scope and, if so, whether those economies will increase or decrease unit costs.

For the purposes of projecting the costs of ART policy, we have adopted the simplifying assumption that most program costs relate to the individual patient—in the form of provider time, pharmaceutical products, diagnostic tests, and disposable paper and rubber products—and therefore do not vary much with scale or scope. The exception we make to this rule is the cost of equipping a health care facility that is not a district hospital with the capacity to administer and manage patients on ART. We assume that to qualify to manage one or more ART patients, any facility must train a minimum number of providers in ART protocols and, to keep them abreast of the rapidly changing technology, must retrain those staff members every year. This category of costs might be called *recurrent fixed costs.* They recur every year as a function of the number of facilities, but they can be spread over all the patients at the facility.

We anticipate that once ART treatment is available at all district hospitals, perhaps by 2008, the government will recognize that expanding coverage requires expanding the number of treatment facilities beyond the district hospital network. One option is to equip a selected number of health centers with a physician and a nurse who are trained in ART. The costs of this additional training and retraining will be repaid with the greater willingness of the population living close to these centers to seek treatment and to adhere to treatment regimens.

## Projection Scenarios

The impact of a policy choice can be defined only in comparison with what would have happened in the absence of the choice. This alternative scenario, called a *baseline* or *counterfactual*, is a projection of the future course of AIDS treatment had the Royal Thai government not introduced its expanded NAPHA. This section describes how the report defines the baseline and the NAPHA scenarios.

### *Baseline and NAPHA Projections*

Several alternative baseline scenarios could have been chosen: cells (a), (b) and (c) in table 4.5. Each scenario corresponds to a different combination of public financing of ART and government subsidization of the production and sale of low-cost ART drugs. The chosen baseline corresponds to cell (a): what would have happened had the government kept only its pre-2001 voluntary program, with only branded drugs available.

The effect of NAPHA is obtained by comparing outcomes from cell (a) with those from cell (d). The total impact can be separated into the part caused by the availability of low-cost generic ART and the part caused by the public finance of ART provision. Such a deconstruction enables us to attribute portions of the benefits of NAPHA to each of its two components and a portion to synergy between them. We do not undertake that deconstruction here.

**Table 4.5**  Potential Baseline Scenarios or Counterfactuals to NAPHA

| | | **Government to finance ART publicly** | |
|---|---|---|---|
| | | *No (private out-of-pocket only)* | *Yes* |
| **Government to produce and sell low-cost ART (GPO-vir)** | *No* | (A) Baseline scenario: No government intervention takes place. There is a voluntary program only, too small to make a difference (for example, no ART). | (B) Government provides subsidized public production with no possibility of alternative supply channels (buyers' clubs and so forth). |
| | *Yes* | (C) GPO produces and markets GPO-vir at current prices (less than US$1/day), but government does not expand public delivery of ART through the public health system beyond the voluntary program. | (D) NAPHA: This scenario includes the current form and alternative versions, including stimulating VCT for earlier recruitment and introducing demand-side incentives to increase adherence. |

*Source:* Authors.

## Assumptions

Table 4.4 categorized the 18 variables, which are generated by the policy model and then drive the epidemiological model. Table 4.6 presents the specific assumptions for the baseline, which characterizes what would have happened had NAPHA not been implemented, and for the changes made by the government, which define the NAPHA policy.

The Thai government implemented the NAPHA policy by changing a number of policy instruments, which in turn affected people's

**Table 4.6** Assumptions for Baseline and NAPHA Scenarios

| | Scenario | | |
| Parameter | Baseline | NAPHA | Change (%) |
|---|---|---|---|
| 1. Price of VCT (baht) | 30 | 30 | 0 |
| 2. Weight of short-run VCT demand in total (%) | 100.0 | 100.0 | 0 |
| 3. Growth rate of VCT facilities (%) | 0.0 | 0.0 | 0 |
| *Prices of ART per year (baht)* | | | |
| 4. Public | 8,530 | 650 | −92.4 |
| 5. Augmented public | 8,530 | 1,880 | −78.0 |
| 6. Private | 13,800 | 9,534 | −30.9 |
| 7. No ART | 30 | 30 | 0 |
| *Quantities of ART in 2003 (number of facilities)* | | | |
| 8. Public | 119 | 860 | 622.7 |
| 9. Augmented public | 45 | 100 | 222.2 |
| 10. Private | 100 | 100 | 0 |
| 11. No ART (residual) | 11,042 | 10,282 | −6.9 |
| *Other ART supply parameters* | | | |
| 12. Growth rate of ART facilities (%) | 1.0 | 1.5 | 50.0 |
| 13. Growth rate of augmented ART facilities (%) | 1.0 | 5.0 | 500.0 |
| 14. Growth rate of private ART facilities (%) | 1.0 | 3.0 | 200.0 |
| 15. Starting number of treatment slots per public facility (average) | 17.6 | 54 | 206.8 |
| 16. Starting number of treatment slots per augmented public facility (average) | 56 | 56 | 0 |
| 17. Proportion of treatment capacity designated to symptomatic patients before asymptomatic patients with CD4 < 200 cells/mm$^3$ are accepted (%) | 90.0 | 90.0 | 0 |
| 18. Growth rate of all public health facilities (%) | 1.0 | 2.0 | 100.0 |
| 19. Number of treatment slots in 2002 | 2,095 | 8,341 | 298.1 |
| 20. Number of treatment slots in 2003 | 2,095 | 16,663 | 695.4 |

*Source:* MOPH data and authors' estimates.

willingness and ability to seek out and use VCT and ART services. Among the most important instruments were the price paid by patients for ART and the distance patients had to travel to obtain it. Table 4.6 shows that the price paid by a patient for ART in a public facility was reduced by 92 percent, and the number of treatment sites was increased more than sixfold, as a result of the NAPHA policy. Because GPO-vir was also available to NGOs and the private sector, the effective prices of treatment fell for those modes of treatment also, though not by as much. We assume that their availability also improved.

Furthermore, in adopting NAPHA, the government launched a process of expansion whose full extent is not yet known. For the purposes of this model, we assume that the number of treatment facilities continues to grow through the end of the projection period by 1.5 percent per year, while the number of patients treated in any given facility expands to meet virtually all available demand. We assume that the NAPHA policy is friendly to but not aggressively promoting the incorporation of PHA groups into the public treatment protocols, so that augmented public treatment grows at 5 percent a year. We assume that private treatment facilities also become increasingly available, with a growth rate of 3 percent a year, though at a substantially higher price.[16]

This model captures our assumptions about the effects of these dramatic policy changes on treatment uptake. Panel (a) of figure 4.7 illustrates the effects on the demand for ART by symptomatic HIV-positive people of the price reduction and the improved availability. Under the 2001 policy, with the price of care at B 8,530 and only 119 facilities delivering care, the proportion of symptomatic AIDS patients nationwide who used care effectively was about 2.4 percent. Another 1 percent of those needing care were being treated in NGOs (that is, the augmented public sector), and we estimate that about 26 percent were being treated in the private sector.[17]

As a result of the reduction in price to B 650 and the increase in availability projected to occur over the next two decades, use will increase for all modes. The second demand curve in panel (a) of figure 4.7 shows the effect of the changes in availability of public ART, while the effect of lower price is shown by moving down from B 8,530 to B 650 on the vertical axis. To enhance the readability of the figure, the price axis is measured on a logarithmic scale. In the new equilibrium

**Figure 4.7** Demand for Public ART as a Function of its Price to the Patient

(a) Demand by symptomatic AIDS patients

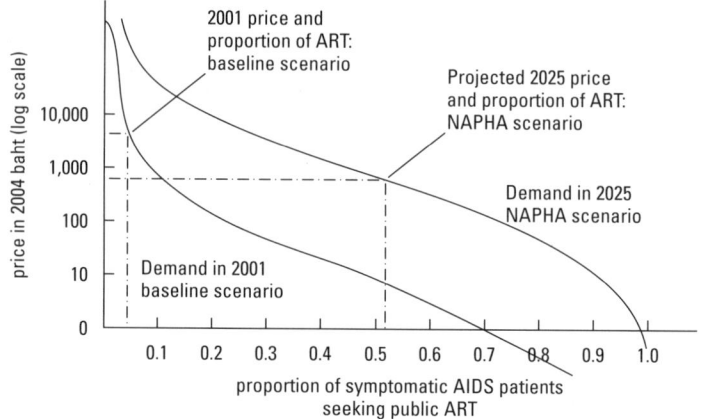

(b) Demand by asymptomatic HIV-positive patients who are informed of their status and eligible for treatment

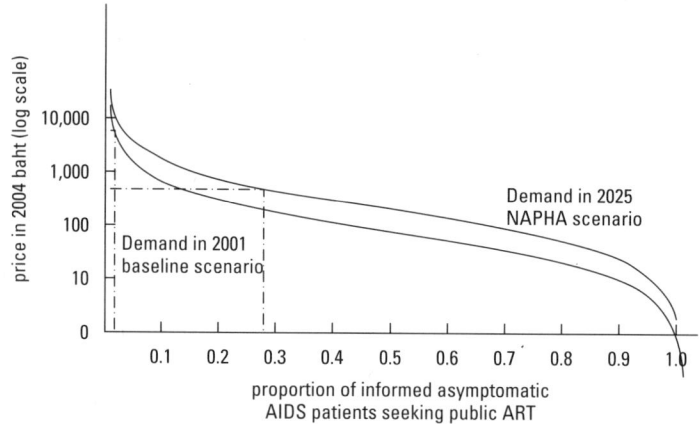

*Source:* Authors.

in 2025 that will result from this combination of policies, 49 percent of the symptomatic AIDS patients will use public sector ART. Another 24 percent will use augmented public or private sector treatment, leaving 27 percent too distant, too poor, or too ill informed to take advantage of public treatment.

Panel (a) can be used to analyze the relative contribution of the price decrease and the availability increase on projected improvements in ART use. According to this demand structure, the price decrease alone would increase ART use only from 0.2 percent to slightly more than 1 percent of symptomatic individuals. Improved availability alone would increase ART use from 0.2 percent to about 20 percent of symptomatic people. However, if this structure is approximately correct, further price decreases by the public sector are likely to increase its share of total AIDS patients, partly at the expense of private care, but partly from among those otherwise unable to afford it.

Panel (b) tells a similar story regarding demand for care among people who are asymptomatic but have tested positive for HIV and are eligible for treatment. The structure of our demand model assumes that because these people typically have much less severe symptoms or no symptoms at all, they are much more responsive to the price of ART. Because they are less sick, they are more able to travel to seek care. So we assume that they are less responsive to improved availability. Reflecting those assumptions, the demand curves for the informed, eligible, asymptomatic are flatter than those for the symptomatic (that is, less price sensitive) and are closer together (showing less effect from the improved availability).

The proportion measured on the horizontal axis of panel (b) in the figure is a fraction of the total number of informed, eligible, asymptomatic, HIV-positive people. According to the structure of the model, for any given point on the asymptomatic demand curve for ART in panel (b), the total number of patients actually recruited depends critically on how many seek testing. Policies that increase the demand for VCT, especially among those at highest risk of infection, increase the number of HIV-positive people who learn of their status and need for treatment early enough to start ART while they are still asymptomatic.

Figure 4.8 presents the demand curves for VCT by the low-risk group and the high-risk group under three scenarios:

- the baseline scenario
- the NAPHA scenario and
- the VCT scenario.[18]

The terms *low-risk* and *high-risk* are composites based on categories of the population in the AEM. Groups from the model that we include in the high-risk aggregate include female sex workers, their clients, men who have sex with men, and IDUs. In the AEM an

**Figure 4.8**  Demand for VCT as a Function of the Price of Public Sector ART: Baseline, NAPHA, and VCT Scenarios

(a) Demand by the high-risk group

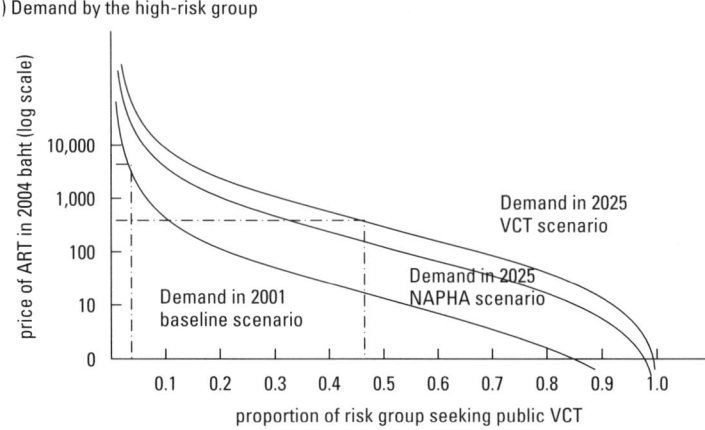

(b) Demand by asymptomatic HIV-positive patients who are informed of their status and eligible for treatment

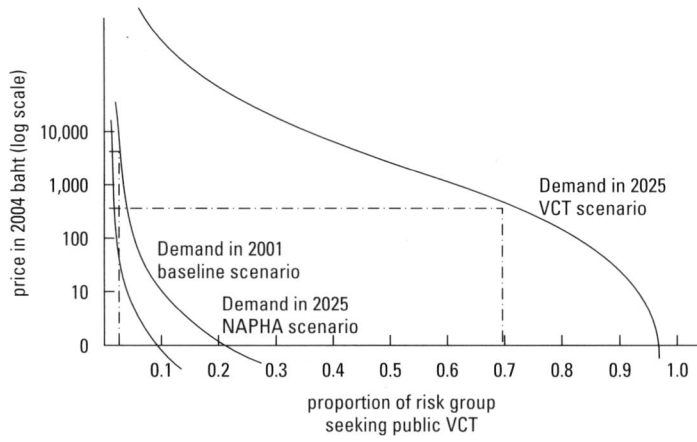

*Source:* Authors.

individual is only temporarily in one of these categories and at higher risk of infection before migrating to another, typically lower-risk category.

We assume the price of VCT remains at B 30 in all the scenarios until the end of the projection period. However, we assume that both the price and the availability of ART affect the demand for VCT. Because ART and VCT are complements in consumption, reductions in the price of ART or improvements in its availability stimulate the demand for VCT. Accordingly, it is useful to construct a demand curve for VCT as a function of the price of ART.

Panel (a) of figure 4.8 shows the effect on the proportion of the high-risk group that demands VCT as a function of the price and availability of ART. The leftmost curve presents the demand structure for 2001, when ART was expensive and only 119 locations offered it. About 2 percent of high-risk people were tested in that year. The second curve shows the effect of improved ART availability under the NAPHA policy as a rightward shift of the demand curve at all ART prices by 2025. The price reduction of public ART from B 8,530 to B 650 is projected to move the equilibrium demand for VCT down that demand curve to a point where about 30 percent of the high-risk group will seek testing.

Panel (b) of figure 4.8 shows the quite different structure of demand for VCT assumed for the low-risk group; it is about 20 times larger than for the high-risk group.[19] The leftmost curve again presents the demand under the baseline scenario, when the price of ART is high and its availability limited. Although the predicted proportion seeking VCT in this group was only about 0.02 percent or about one-tenth as large as in the high-risk group, the absolute number of low-risk people tested would have been almost twice as large as the number of high-risk people tested in 2001. Because HIV prevalence in 2001 was slightly less than 1 percent among low-risk adults and more than 4 percent among high-risk adults, the high-risk group would still have more positive tests. For 2001, we estimate about 3,600 positive test results among asymptomatic people, of which about 2,600 were in high-risk groups.

Because low-risk people may not perceive themselves to be in danger of infection, we model their demand for testing as more sensitive to the price and availability of VCT than to the price and availability of ART. The leftmost two demand curves in panel (b) are steep to represent this lack of responsiveness (or inelasticity) with respect to the price of ART. Furthermore, when the NAPHA policy improves ART availability by 2025, the demand curve shifts only a small amount to the right.[20] The total increase in the proportion of low-risk people seeking VCT in the NAPHA scenario is from 0.2 percent to 1.8 percent. Although this increase is almost tenfold, this small demand suggests that without strong and dramatic new policy measures only a very small minority of the general population will learn their HIV status.

The policy model generates the percentage of people in each risk group who will seek VCT and the proportional distribution of asymptomatic and symptomatic patients across the four treatment modes in each year of the progression period. Figure 4.9 presents these three projections for the baseline situation in 2001 and for the NAPHA scenario in 2025.

This section has shown how the policy model links changes in the policy instruments to changes in the distribution of demand for VCT and ART. These proportional distributions are then provided as input to drive the AEM. The next section examines the health and financial consequences of these inputs in the context of the epidemiological and demographic structure of the Thai epidemic.

### Effects of Current Policy (NAPHA)

The discussion in the previous section makes clear how dramatic was the change in Thai AIDS treatment policy in 2002.[21] Over just a few months, the price of publicly provided ART dropped by 92 percent, and its availability soared by 620 percent. Because of the new lower price of generically produced ART medications, even the price of private sector ART declined by 30 percent. In this context, projecting the course of the current NAPHA policy is a somewhat arbitrary exercise. We assume that the number of facilities continues to grow at 1.5 percent a year, and we allow the number of persons treated per facility to grow to accommodate all the demand that is elicited by the resulting decrease in the average distance of people from facilities.

Under these assumptions, figure 4.10 demonstrates the result that was predicted in early chapters: by keeping people alive, the NAPHA policy (including second-line therapy) increases the number of HIV-infected people in Thailand compared with what it would have been in the absence of treatment. The model predicts that by 2025 the number of HIV-infected adults will be four times larger than it would have been without NAPHA (263,000 instead of 62,000). Most of this increase occurs because people who would have died of AIDS are living much longer, but some of it is due to increased transmission of HIV by people who are living longer with HIV infection.[22]

Figure 4.11 shows the effect of NAPHA with second-line therapy on the path of annual total adult deaths in Thailand. A sharp reduction in deaths can be seen at the start of the program—the result of a large cohort of HIV-infected people beginning treatment and surviving

**Figure 4.9** Projected Effects of the NAPHA Policy on Demand for VCT and ART

(a) Poportion of low- and high-risk groups seeking VCT in baseline and NAPHA scenarios.

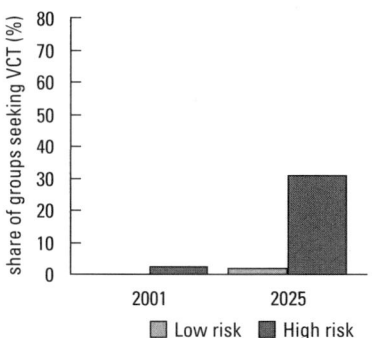

(b) Proportion of asymptomatic patients seeking ART in baseline and NAPHA scenarios.

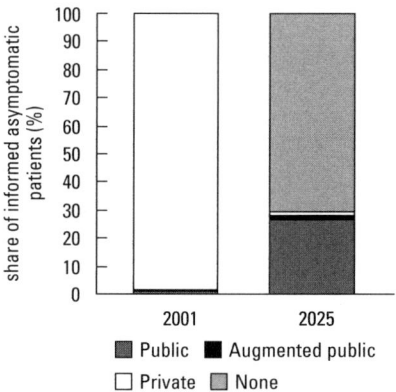

(c) Proportion of symptomatic patients seeking ART in baseline and NAPHA scenarios.

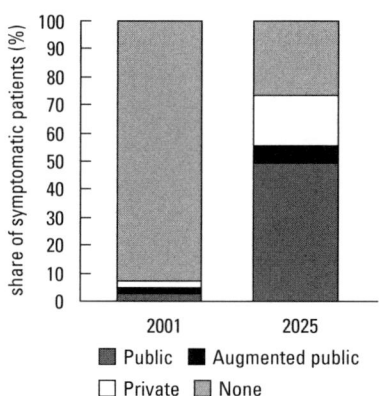

*Source:* Authors.

**Figure 4.10** Projected Current HIV Cases

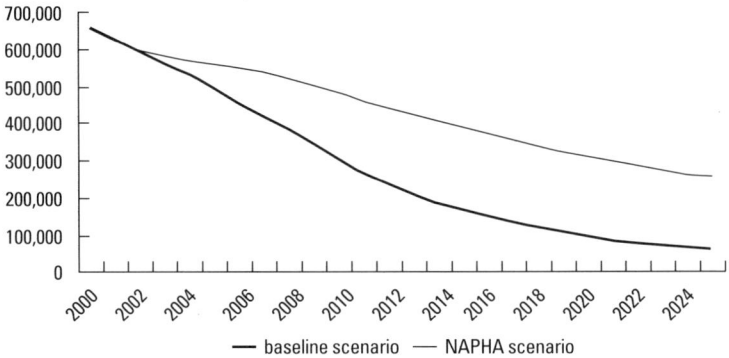

*Source:* Authors.

longer. Figure 4.11 also reveals why "deaths averted" is not a good measure of the success of the ART program. By preventing the deaths of many AIDS patients beginning in 2002, NAPHA postpones those deaths about 12 years. When the patients eventually begin to die, total deaths rebound upward until, in 2017, they exceed the number who would have died that year without NAPHA. The considerable achievement of NAPHA is to shift the survival distribution of AIDS patients to longer survival times, so that the average AIDS patient lives between 5 and 15 years longer. Because everyone dies eventually, the additional deaths after 2017 are not a negative consequence of the program, but a reflection of the longer survival times of the patients.

**Figure 4.11** Projected Annual AIDS Deaths

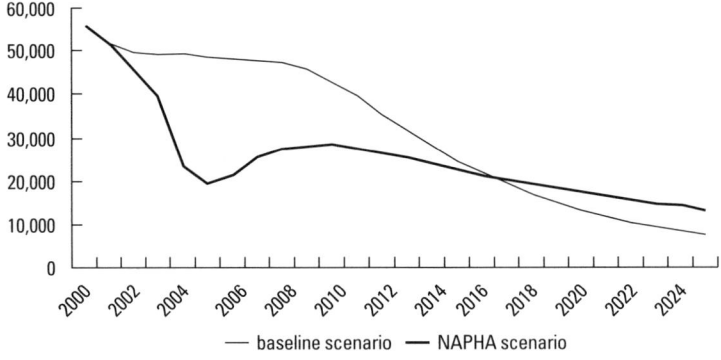

*Source:* Authors.

The cumulating number of patients under treatment has direct implications for the treatment burden on the health sector. Figure 4.12 shows the extraordinary increase in the national treatment burden attributable to NAPHA with second-line therapy. Under the model's assumptions regarding the benefits of treatment and the declining incidence of new HIV cases, the number of PHAs on treatment under NAPHA peaks in 2015 at about 230,000 and then begins to decrease slowly. Unlike the vast majority of Thai patients, these chronic AIDS patients will have ongoing relationships with the public health system that will last a decade or more. To provide and sustain high-quality care, the system will have to develop and apply modern methods of handling patient records at all the hundreds of treatment sites. Through repeated experience with the health care system, patients will become increasingly informed and thus increasingly likely to point out deficiencies they perceive. So the task of managing communications with this growing patient population will increase in importance from both a medical and a political perspective.

As a measure of the direct benefits of an ART provision policy we use the number of life-years saved, computed as the number of additional people alive in any given year.[23,24] Figure 4.13 presents the predicted flow of saved life-years that result from the implementation of NAPHA with second-line therapy. This figure illustrates the dramatic benefits achieved through the NAPHA policy. By 2015, it will have added about 220,000 people to the living population. Even at the end of the projection horizon, when the Thai AIDS epidemic is predicted to be less severe, the NAPHA policy will save about 190,000 life-years each year.

**Figure 4.12**   Projected Number of HIV-Positive People on ART

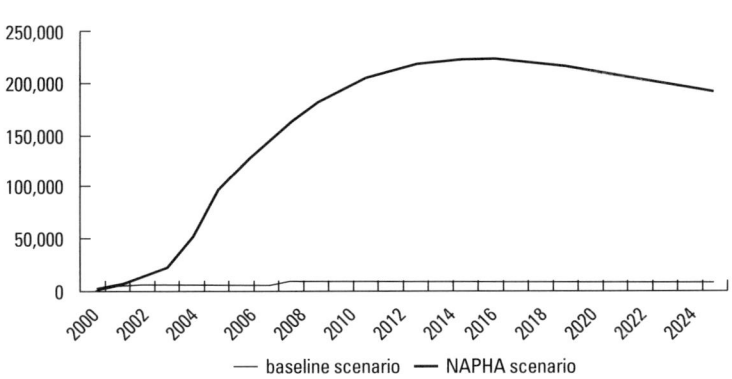

*Source:* Authors.

**Figure 4.13**  Projected Annual Flow of Life-Years Saved under NAPHA

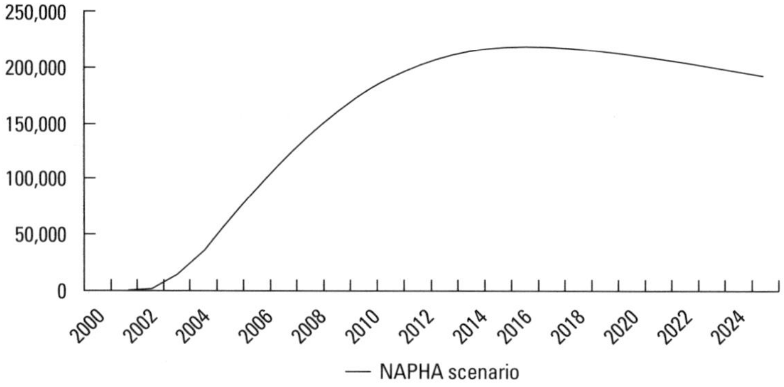

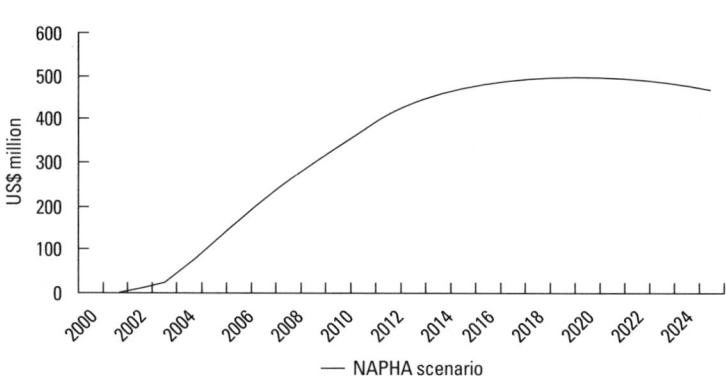

*Source:* Authors.

## Costs and Cost-Effectiveness of Current Policy

What are the budget implications of the NAPHA policy, and can the Thai government afford them? To answer those questions, we apply the cost structure described above to the baseline scenario (A) and the NAPHA scenario (D1).

### *Projected Costs (Baseline and NAPHA)*

Figure 4.14 displays the financial implications of the NAPHA policy with second-line therapy compared with those of the baseline. We project costs in millions of U.S. dollars and show that they soon attain

**Figure 4.14**  Projected Net Costs of ART under NAPHA

*Source:* Authors.

a sum more than 30 times the cost of the baseline scenario. Projected costs of ART are the net costs, which add the costs of ART drugs, other hospital services, VCT, and the net cost of treating opportunistic illnesses. These net cost computations subtract the forgone costs of treatment of those illnesses at the beginning of ART and then add those costs back to the total when treatment fails. Costs will peak in 2019 at US$500 million in 2004 dollars (B 20 billion) per year before leveling off.

Figure 4.15 breaks the total cost of public ART in the NAPHA scenario into four components:

- symptomatic patients in first-line therapy

- symptomatic patients in second-line therapy

- asymptomatic patients in first-line therapy

- asymptomatic patients in second-line therapy.

Beginning in 2010, expenditures on second-line therapy generate more than half the cost of treatment. By the end of the projection, second-line therapy for one-fourth of all the patients are responsible for three-fourths of the treatment budget (figure 4.16).

**Figure 4.15**  Projected Total Cost of Public ART under NAPHA by Line of Treatment

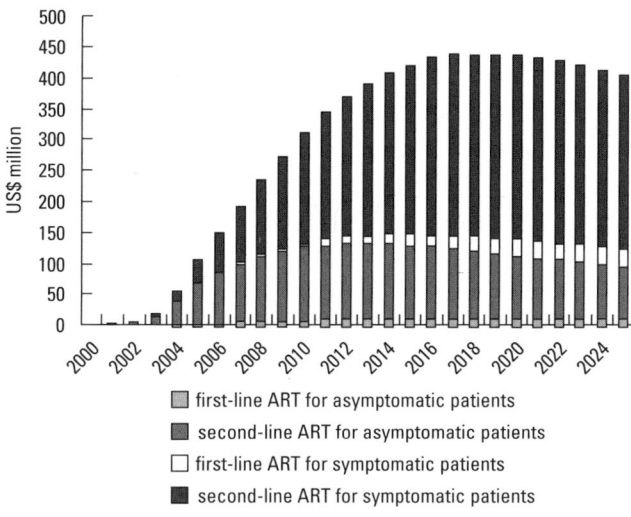

*Source:* Authors.

**Figure 4.16**  Percentage of Total Cost of NAPHA Attributable to Second-Line ART

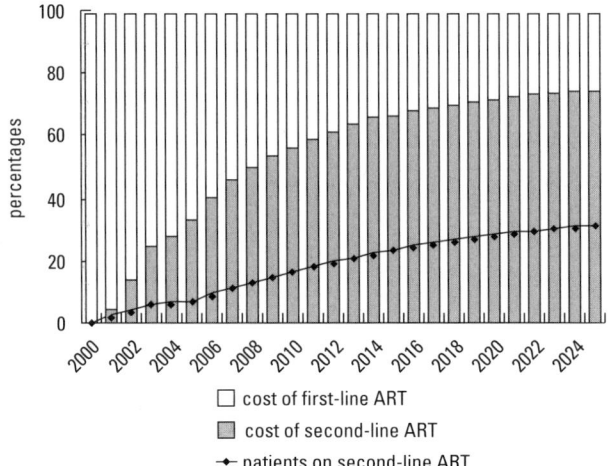

Source: Authors.

As explained above, these projections assume constant future prices. Of course, if the price of second-line treatment falls as much as the price of first-line treatment has fallen, the cost of second-line treatment—and thus the overall costs—will be greatly reduced. However, ongoing World Trade Organization negotiations and bilateral negotiations between the United States and countries such as Brazil, China, South Africa, and Thailand are tending to strengthen patent protection regimes for all drugs. Accordingly, in these simulations, we keep drug prices unchanged throughout the projection period. In chapter 6, we analyze the sensitivity of the cost projections and the cost-effectiveness results to various alternative assumptions, including the possibility of low-cost second-line drugs.

### Financial Implications of NAPHA

The calculations above project the annual incremental cost of the NAPHA program to the Thai government.[25] Cost projections show that under the NAPHA policy as modeled here, costs increase sharply, tripling current ART expenditures in a few years. The trend of rapid growth continues until 2020, when total expenditure levels off at close to US$500 million in 2004 dollars (B 40 billion) per year. The present value of the future stream of additional expenditures engendered by

NAPHA totals US$5.6 billion or B 226.4 billion through 2025 in 2004 dollars.

Will expenditures of this magnitude be affordable for Thailand? *Affordable* has no precise economic definition. Affordability is ultimately a political judgment of whether relevant stakeholders will tolerate a given level of spending. However, in almost any country, a sudden and dramatic increase in the amount and proportion of government spending devoted to a single disease requires justification. The cost increases charted in the previous section are certainly sudden and dramatic by any standard.

Tables 4.7 and 4.8 compare those projected future expenditures with the projected levels of the AIDS budget and the total health budget, assuming those two budgets grow at a constant 5.2 percent per year in real terms. In 2004, the net cost of ART under the NAPHA program was estimated at US$77.3 million (B 3,000), 26 percent more than was originally budgeted for AIDS that year and 6.5 percent of the national health budget. From consuming about 1 percent of the health budget and about a third of the AIDS budget in 2001, the public cost of AIDS treatment is projected to rise by 2013 to almost one-fourth of the entire health budget and about seven times the projected (constant growth) AIDS budget. Subsequently costs grow more slowly, so that by 2025 the cost of ART will be about four times the constant growth AIDS budget and about 13.5 percent of the projected health budget.

In addition to general revenue, Thailand has two other sources of revenue to finance the rapidly increasing cost of ART. First, the Global Fund to Fight AIDS, Tuberculosis, and Malaria (GFATM) has already granted the country US$200 million (B 8 billion) for the next few years, of which US$13.5 million (B 540 million) is designated for the MOPH, to cover the cost of the ART program in 2004. Second, several national health insurance schemes—the Universal Coverage Scheme (UCS); the Social Security Scheme for formal sector workers; and the Civil Service Medical Benefit Scheme—are also a source of financing for PHA care, including ART. In 2001, Thailand achieved universal coverage of health care by extending insurance coverage through the UCS. As of 2004, the UCS covers the costs of treatment of opportunistic infections, some lab tests, and hospital services (except the costs of antiretroviral drugs for ART patients, which are

**Table 4.7**  Projected Costs of the NAPHA Policy for ART, Including Second-Line Therapy, 2001–25

|  | 2000 | 2001 | 2002 | 2003 | 2004 | 2005 | 2006 | 2007 | 2008 | 2009 | 2010 | 2011 | 2012 |
|---|---|---|---|---|---|---|---|---|---|---|---|---|---|
| *Baseline* | | | | | | | | | | | | | |
| Net cost of ART | — | 10.7 | 11.4 | 12.4 | 12.5 | 12.4 | 12.4 | 12.4 | 12.4 | 12.2 | 12.0 | 11.6 | 11.1 |
| First-line ART cost | — | 3.3 | 4.0 | 4.2 | 4.3 | 4.3 | 4.3 | 4.4 | 4.4 | 4.5 | 4.6 | 4.7 | 4.7 |
| Second-line ART cost | — | 0.4 | 0.6 | 0.8 | 0.8 | 0.8 | 0.8 | 0.8 | 0.8 | 0.7 | 0.7 | 0.7 | 0.7 |
| Share of second-line cost (%) | — | 3.5 | 5.6 | 6.1 | 6.3 | 6.3 | 6.3 | 6.2 | 6.1 | 6.1 | 6.2 | 6.4 | 6.6 |
| Share of people on second-line ART (%) | — | 1.6 | 2.2 | 2.3 | 2.5 | 2.5 | 2.5 | 2.4 | 2.4 | 2.3 | 2.3 | 2.2 | 2.2 |
| *NAPHA policy* | | | | | | | | | | | | | |
| Net cost of ART | — | 10.9 | 19.2 | 33.3 | 77.3 | 130.8 | 176.8 | 224.0 | 270.5 | 314.8 | 355.4 | 391.2 | 421.9 |
| First-line ART cost | — | 3.3 | 10.3 | 18.9 | 46.4 | 78.8 | 96.6 | 112.0 | 125.0 | 135.5 | 143.2 | 148.0 | 150.5 |
| Second-line ART cost | — | 0.5 | 2.7 | 8.3 | 21.6 | 43.3 | 71.1 | 102.4 | 135.5 | 169.0 | 201.8 | 232.7 | 260.9 |
| Share of second-line cost (%) | — | 4.8 | 14.3 | 24.8 | 27.9 | 33.1 | 40.2 | 45.7 | 50.1 | 53.7 | 56.8 | 59.5 | 61.9 |
| Share of people on second-line ART (%) | — | 2.3 | 3.7 | 5.9 | 6.3 | 6.9 | 9.1 | 11.1 | 13.0 | 14.7 | 16.4 | 18.0 | 19.5 |

**Table 4.7** Continued

| | 2013 | 2014 | 2015 | 2016 | 2017 | 2018 | 2019 | 2020 | 2021 | 2022 | 2023 | 2024 | 2025 |
|---|---|---|---|---|---|---|---|---|---|---|---|---|---|
| *Baseline* | | | | | | | | | | | | | |
| Net cost of ART | 10.7 | 10.3 | 9.9 | 9.6 | 9.4 | 9.1 | 8.8 | 8.5 | 8.2 | 7.9 | 7.5 | 7.3 | 7.0 |
| First-line ART cost | 4.8 | 4.9 | 5.0 | 5.1 | 5.1 | 5.1 | 5.1 | 5.1 | 5.0 | 4.8 | 4.7 | 4.6 | 4.4 |
| Second-line ART cost | 0.7 | 0.7 | 0.7 | 0.7 | 0.7 | 0.7 | 0.7 | 0.7 | 0.7 | 0.6 | 0.6 | 0.6 | 0.5 |
| Share of second-line cost (%) | 6.9 | 7.2 | 7.4 | 7.7 | 7.9 | 8.1 | 8.2 | 8.3 | 8.3 | 8.3 | 8.1 | 8.0 | 7.8 |
| Share of people on second-line ART (%) | 2.2 | 2.1 | 2.1 | 2.1 | 2.0 | 2.0 | 2.0 | 2.0 | 1.9 | 1.9 | 1.9 | 1.8 | 1.8 |
| *NAPHA policy* | | | | | | | | | | | | | |
| Net cost of ART | 447.3 | 467.7 | 483.4 | 494.8 | 502.4 | 506.7 | 508.1 | 507.0 | 503.8 | 498.9 | 492.7 | 485.3 | 477.0 |
| First-line ART cost | 151.0 | 150.1 | 148.1 | 145.3 | 142.0 | 138.4 | 134.5 | 130.6 | 126.6 | 122.6 | 118.8 | 115.0 | 111.4 |
| Second-line ART cost | 285.9 | 307.3 | 325.0 | 339.3 | 350.2 | 358.2 | 363.4 | 366.3 | 367.1 | 366.1 | 363.7 | 360.0 | 355.3 |
| Share of second-line cost (%) | 63.9 | 65.7 | 67.2 | 68.6 | 69.7 | 70.7 | 71.5 | 72.2 | 72.9 | 73.4 | 73.8 | 74.2 | 74.5 |
| Share of people on second-line ART (%) | 20.9 | 22.2 | 23.5 | 24.6 | 25.6 | 26.6 | 27.4 | 28.2 | 28.9 | 29.6 | 30.2 | 30.7 | 31.2 |

*Source:* Authors.
*Note:* All monetary values are in millions of 2004 US dollars. — = not available.

127

**Table 4.8** Projected Costs of the NAPHA Policy for ART, Including Second-Line Therapy, as Percentage of AIDS Budget and Health Budget, 2001–25

| | 2000 | 2001 | 2002 | 2003 | 2004 | 2005 | 2006 | 2007 | 2008 | 2009 | 2010 | 2011 | 2012 |
|---|---|---|---|---|---|---|---|---|---|---|---|---|---|
| *Baseline* | | | | | | | | | | | | | |
| Net cost of ART | — | 10.7 | 11.4 | 12.4 | 12.5 | 12.4 | 12.4 | 12.4 | 12.4 | 12.2 | 12.0 | 11.6 | 11.1 |
| AIDS budget | — | 37.2 | 36.8 | 29.7 | 61.4 | 67.2 | 69.5 | 71.8 | 49.9 | 52.5 | 55.2 | 58.1 | 61.1 |
| Health budget | — | 1,130.7 | 1,130.7 | 1,130.7 | 1,190.6 | 1,253.7 | 1,320.1 | 1,390.1 | 1,463.8 | 1,541.3 | 1,623.0 | 1,709.1 | 1,799.6 |
| Share of AIDS budget (%) | — | 28.9 | 31.0 | 41.7 | 20.3 | 18.5 | 17.9 | 17.3 | 24.8 | 23.3 | 21.8 | 20.0 | 18.2 |
| Share of health budget (%) | — | 0.9 | 1.0 | 1.1 | 1.0 | 1.0 | 0.9 | 0.9 | 0.8 | 0.8 | 0.7 | 0.7 | 0.6 |
| *NAPHA policy* | | | | | | | | | | | | | |
| Net cost of ART | — | 10.9 | 19.2 | 33.3 | 77.3 | 130.8 | 176.8 | 224.0 | 270.5 | 314.8 | 355.4 | 391.2 | 421.9 |
| AIDS budget | — | 37.2 | 36.8 | 29.7 | 61.4 | 67.2 | 69.5 | 71.8 | 49.9 | 52.5 | 55.2 | 58.1 | 61.1 |
| Health budget | — | 1,130.7 | 1,130.7 | 1,130.7 | 1,190.6 | 1,253.7 | 1,320.1 | 1,390.1 | 1,463.8 | 1,541.3 | 1,623.0 | 1,709.1 | 1,799.6 |
| Share of AIDS budget (%) | — | 29.2 | 52.1 | 112.1 | 125.9 | 194.6 | 254.5 | 312.0 | 542.1 | 599.6 | 643.5 | 673.3 | 690.2 |
| Share of health budget (%) | — | 1.0 | 1.7 | 2.9 | 6.5 | 10.4 | 13.4 | 16.1 | 18.5 | 20.4 | 21.9 | 22.9 | 23.4 |

**Table 4.8** Continued

| | 2013 | 2014 | 2015 | 2016 | 2017 | 2018 | 2019 | 2020 | 2021 | 2022 | 2023 | 2024 | 2025 |
|---|---|---|---|---|---|---|---|---|---|---|---|---|---|
| *Baseline* | | | | | | | | | | | | | |
| Net cost of ART | 10.7 | 10.3 | 9.9 | 9.6 | 9.4 | 9.1 | 8.8 | 8.5 | 8.2 | 7.9 | 7.5 | 7.3 | 7.0 |
| AIDS budget | 64.3 | 67.6 | 71.2 | 74.9 | 78.8 | 82.8 | 87.2 | 91.7 | 96.5 | 101.5 | 106.7 | 112.3 | 118.1 |
| Health budget | 1,895.0 | 1,995.4 | 2,101.2 | 2,212.6 | 2,329.8 | 2,453.3 | 2,583.3 | 2,720.3 | 2,864.4 | 3,016.2 | 3,176.1 | 3,344.4 | 3,521.7 |
| Share of AIDS budget (%) | 16.6 | 15.2 | 14.0 | 12.9 | 11.9 | 10.9 | 10.1 | 9.3 | 8.5 | 7.7 | 7.1 | 6.5 | 5.9 |
| Share of health budget (%) | 0.6 | 0.5 | 0.5 | 0.4 | 0.4 | 0.4 | 0.3 | 0.3 | 0.3 | 0.3 | 0.2 | 0.2 | 0.2 |
| *NAPHA policy* | | | | | | | | | | | | | |
| Net cost of ART | 447.3 | 467.7 | 483.4 | 494.8 | 502.4 | 506.7 | 508.1 | 507.0 | 503.8 | 498.9 | 492.7 | 485.3 | 477.0 |
| AIDS budget | 64.3 | 67.6 | 71.2 | 74.9 | 78.8 | 82.8 | 87.2 | 91.7 | 96.5 | 101.5 | 106.7 | 112.3 | 118.1 |
| Health budget | 1,895.0 | 1,995.4 | 2,101.2 | 2,212.6 | 2,329.8 | 2,453.3 | 2,583.3 | 2,720.3 | 2,864.4 | 3,016.2 | 3,176.1 | 3,344.4 | 3,521.7 |
| Share of AIDS budget (%) | 695.6 | 691.4 | 679.3 | 660.9 | 638.0 | 611.6 | 582.9 | 552.9 | 522.3 | 491.7 | 461.5 | 432.1 | 403.7 |
| Share of health budget (%) | 23.6 | 23.4 | 23.0 | 22.4 | 21.6 | 20.7 | 19.7 | 18.6 | 17.6 | 16.5 | 15.5 | 14.5 | 13.5 |

*Source:* Authors.

*Note:* All monetary values are in millions of 2004 US dollars. An annual growth rate of 5.2 percent is assumed for the AIDS budget, health budget, and public health spending from 2004 to 2025, on the basis of 2004 figures. AIDS budgets during 2004 and 2008 include first and second round allocations from the Global Fund for AIDS, Tuberculosis, and Malaria.

covered by NAPHA), with a nominal fee of less than US$0.80 per visit (B 30). The Social Security Scheme covers treatment of opportunistic infections and, since August 2004, also the cost of ART (with caps) for its affiliated members (but not for their families). The Civil Service Medical Benefit Scheme covers all care for PHAs including ART (see chapter 2).

Although the projection shows a significant increase in ART expenditure over time, it remains less than 24 percent of the (constant growth) national health budget. Because a reduction of more than 20 percent in other health expenditures is unlikely, Thailand can finance these additional expenditures from such outside sources as the GFATM and health insurance schemes, or it can increase the size of the overall health budget as a share of total government spending.

### Cost-Effectiveness of NAPHA

Figure 4.17 presents the model's projections of the annual benefits and the annual costs of the NAPHA policy, compared with the baseline scenario of limited public sector access to ART. The annual benefits measured in life-years saved increase rapidly, peaking in 2017. These benefits begin to level off as the stock of AIDS patients gradually declines. Because of the slow transition of patients to the more expensive second-line therapy, costs continue rising, peaking at about US$500 million (B 20 billion) in 2020 before leveling off.

**Figure 4.17**  Benefit (Life-Years Saved) and Costs of NAPHA Relative to Baseline

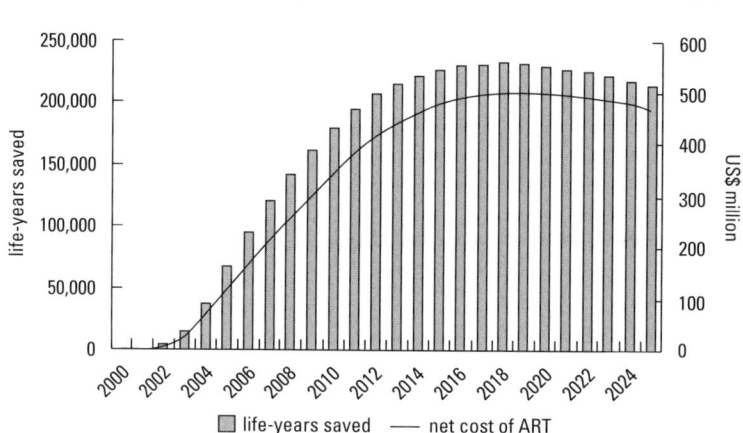

life-years saved ▪ life-years saved  —— net cost of ART

*Source:* Authors.

When the benefits of any intervention occur relatively soon after the program is launched and costs occur later, discounting reduces the importance of the future costs in relation to the near-term benefits and thus improves the cost-effectiveness of the program. Figure 4.18 presents the net present value of the cost per life-year saved for the NAPHA policy, with all costs and benefits discounted back to 2002. The choice of discount rate has a small but significant effect on the result. At a zero discount rate, the NAPHA program costs close to US$2,200 (B 88,000) per life-year saved, whereas at a 15 percent discount rate, the cost of the same life-year saved would be US$2,000 (B 8,000). At the conventional discount rate of 3 percent, the cost per life-year saved for the NAPHA policy is US$2,145 (B 85,800), slightly greater than Thailand's 2002 gross national income per capita of US$2,000 (B 80,000).

Is US$2,145 (B 85,800) a large or a small price for the Thai government to pay to save years of life through a special treatment subsidy program? Different observers have differing views. An argument for horizontal equity would ask whether the government is willing to pay as much to buy life-years through subsidized treatment of other adult illnesses, such as cancer, heart disease, or end-stage renal disease. Advocates of vertical equity would point out that this sum is small enough to make treatment a good personal investment for people in

**Figure 4.18**  Cost Effectiveness of NAPHA at Different Discount Rates

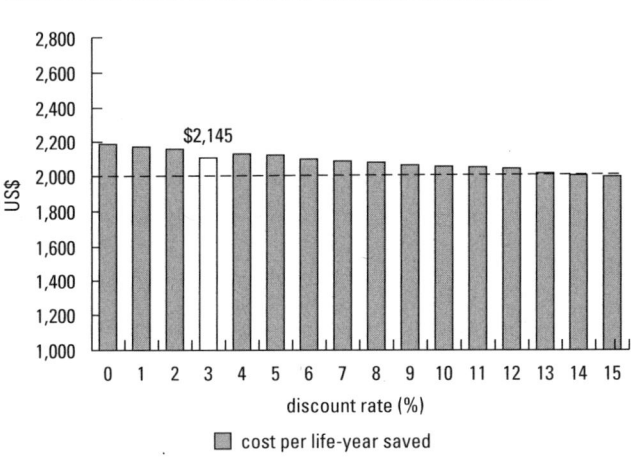

*Source:* Authors.

the upper quintile of Thailand's income distribution, where incomes per capita exceed US$10,000 (B 400,000). Therefore, in the interest of vertical equity, the government should ensure that people in the bottom four-fifths of the income distribution have access to care that the those in the top one-fifth will purchase for themselves. Before entering further into this discussion (in chapter 6), we turn to the question of how modifications of NAPHA will affect its benefits and costs, possibly improving its attractiveness as a health policy.

## Notes

1. Christianson (1976) is one of the earliest examples. See the other sources cited for applications in a development context. None of these authors considers the demand for diagnostic information as a precursor to the demand for care, as we do in the discussion of figure 4.2.

2. In microeconomic theory, this assumption is referred to as homotheticity and is frequently adopted to improve the tractability of economic models of demand.

3. McFadden (1974) first used the conditional multinomial logit specification to model the commuters' choice between bus, car, and train modes of transportation in the San Francisco Bay area.

4. Note that the numerator of the multinomial logit demand function is an exponential function of price and distance. Exponential functions are always positive. Further note that the denominator of the demand function is the sum of the numerators for the four modes. Hence, by the choice of this functional form, each mode demand is guaranteed to be a positive fraction between zero and one, and the sum of the four demand functions is guaranteed to equal one.

5. To see this relationship, one may note that according to the functional form, the logarithm of the ratio of two proportions—say public and augmented public—can be written as a linear function of the logarithms of the price and distance ratios between the same two options: $LN(q\_pub\_art/q\_apub\_art) = (\alpha\_pub - \alpha\_apub) + \beta * LN(P\_pub\_art/P\_apub\_art) - \gamma * LN(D\_pub\_art/D\_apub\_art)$.

6. Economists refer to a demand sensitivity such as this, where the response is smaller than the stimulus, as inelastic. In microeconomic studies of the demand for acute medical care, patients have typically been found to be inelastic to price, with elasticities of –0.2 or even closer to zero. We have chosen a value less close to zero because we are modeling the behavior of a population that is on average quite poor and therefore can be expected to be more sensitive to price.

7. When a lower price for one good increases the demand not only for it but also for another good, the two goods are said to be complements in consumption.

8. We consider that every HIV-negative adult has a probability of seeking VCT in any given year.

9. This is the meaning of the term semiempirical, which the published papers use to describe the model.

10. Although sometimes referred to as migration, the behavior captured by these assumptions primarily concerns sexual behavior rather than geographic migration. In the case of sex workers, the transition out of sex work may often be accompanied by a physical change of location, such as a return to a rural hometown. The AEM does not attempt to model geographic location or movements.

11. An example of the difference equations that are the building blocks of the model is the expression for new infections among male clients (Thai Working Group on HIV/AIDS Projection 2001).

12. The figure is not large enough to display the full structure for both early and late treatment. The reader is asked to imagine the same structure for late treatment as is displayed for early treatment.

13. Because we generally assume that Thai policy on the availability of ART will accommodate demand, this constraint on treatment slots is rarely binding in the model runs presented here.

14. The study of the costs and effects of AIDS treatment in India by Over and others (2004) presents the discounted averted years of

orphanhood estimated to result from the simulated alternative policies. However, it eschews the attempt to aggregate these benefits with the benefits of healthy life-years saved.

15.   The rate of discount is much less certain than the fact that discounting is necessary. One golden rule is that costs and effects should be discounted at the same discount rate. However, the best choice for that rate is not clear. This report follows the lead of the 1993 World Development Report on health in adopting a discount rate of 3 percent.

16.   We assume that the private sector will serve only symptomatic patients. Although not strictly correct, this assumption may approximate reality to the extent that demand by the asymptomatic is more price elastic.

17.   The augmented public and private sector demands are not shown in the figure.

18.   Here we discuss the baseline and NAPHA scenarios, returning in the next section to the VCT scenario.

19.   AEM baseline data show approximately 46 million low-risk adults in 2001 and about 2.6 million high-risk adults.

20.   The far right demand curve in panel (b) illustrates the effect of the expanded VCT scenario, discussed in chapter 5.

21.   This section draws on Masaki (2004).

22.   We assume that HIV-infected people under treatment are 75 percent less infectious on each sexual contact than they would have been without ART. Chapter 6 performs sensitivity analysis with respect to this assumption.

23.   In a real population, this measure would be increased by both the number of people who are living longer because of effective ART and also by the fertility of those people. However, the AEM does not model

fertility. Instead it grows the population by adding a new 15-year-old cohort of people every year, whose size is independent of the size of the current population. Therefore, the difference between two scenarios in the size of the population in any year is due entirely to differences in ART.

24. We do not adjust life-years for the degree of disability as was done in computing the disability adjusted life-years burden of disease in the 1993 World Development Report (World Bank 1993).

25. This section is based on Masaki (2004).

# CHAPTER 5

# Policies to Strengthen Treatment Programs: Evaluating the Costs and Benefits of Alternative Policy Scenarios

The assumptions used to project the future of the NAPHA (National Access to Antiretrovirals Program for People Living with AIDS) policy represent a minimal, least-cost approach to meeting the political mandate of the Ministry of Public Health (MOPH) to make treatment available to all. However, more could be done to improve treatment in several ways. Moreover, some of these additional expenditures, though increasing the complexity and cost of antiretroviral therapy (ART) policy, might improve its effectiveness at low enough cost to be worthwhile from a cost-effectiveness perspective.

## Alternative ART Policy Scenarios

In addition to the NAPHA policy scenario described in chapter 4, the report considers two enhancements to NAPHA and a third policy that combines these two enhancements (table 5.1). The enhancements address what are perceived by knowledgeable Thai and international observers to be potential weak points in NAPHA and, indeed, in all publicly financed and provided ART programs worldwide.

Early analyses of the effectiveness and cost-effectiveness of publicly provided ART assumed that many HIV-infected patients would be recruited to treatment when their immune systems first dropped below an eligibility threshold (usually CD4 counts less than 200 to

**Table 5.1**  Typology of Four Major Policy Alternatives for ART Policy Scenarios for the NAPHA program

| | | *Encourage VCT and early recruitment into ART* | |
|---|---|---|---|
| Encourage adherence through demand-side incentives such as PHA groups, accompagnateurs, and conditional transfers | | *No* | *Yes* |
| | *No* | NAPHA (D1): Current implementation of NAPHA (recruit mainly symptomatic HIV-infected persons through the public health system) | VCT (D2): Earlier recruitment through VCT of people at higher CD4 counts, without improved adherence |
| | *Yes* | Adherence (D3): Improved adherence without earlier recruitment (keep current recruitment of symptomatic HIV-infected persons through the public health system) | VCT and adherence (D4): Improved adherence and earlier recruitment (recruit earlier through VCT of persons with higher CD4 counts) |

*Source:* Authors.

250 cubic millimeters so that the benefits of ART would be maximized. However, experiences in Thailand as well as in several other countries—such as Botswana, Brazil, Malawi, and countries of the Organisation for Economic Co-operation and Development (OECD)—show that the vast majority of patients are identified as eligible for ART only when their opportunistic infections lead them to the hospital, when their CD4 counts are already well below the threshold at which they would most benefit from care (see chapter 3). It is thus useful to analyze an alternative version of NAPHA that includes much more vigorous promotion of voluntary counseling and testing (VCT) in an effort to attract patients into treatment when they first become eligible for it. The column labeled VCT (D2) in table 5.2 presents the parameter values used to capture this policy in the policy model. By lowering the price of VCT and increasing its accessibility, the government would elicit more demand for VCT.[1] Among those tested, some would find they are HIV positive; some of those would have CD4 counts low enough to be eligible for treatment. Our VCT scenario (D2) estimates the costs and effects of this alternative version of the NAPHA policy in relation to both the baseline and the basic NAPHA scenario (D1).

A major challenge for ART programs is to attain and sustain high levels of adherence among patients. MOPH-sponsored training programs for public sector ART providers are currently teaching the importance of adherence. But experience around the world suggests that as ART treatment is scaled up, it is increasingly difficult to attain high levels of adherence among new patients and to sustain them among all patients. One promising approach with which Thailand has already experimented is to subsidize and to facilitate the organization of nongovernmental organizations (NGOs) that provide emotional, physical, and sometimes even financial support to patients. In this report, we refer to public sector delivery that has been strengthened by the addition of these demand-enhancing programs as *augmented*. Our augmented scenario (D3) is intended to capture the incremental benefits and costs of such a program.

We also model a program we call *both* (D4), which includes the costs of both expanded VCT and augmented adherence and models a synergistic benefit between them. The typology of these policy alternatives is presented in table 5.1 and their parameter values are given in table 5.2.

The major change introduced into the parameter list to capture the VCT scenario (D2) is an increased rate of growth of VCT. Instead of remaining constant, as in the NAPHA scenario, the number of VCT centers grows at 15 percent per year. In the augmented scenario (D3), VCT numbers remain constant but public sector facilities transform rapidly (at 20 percent per year) from offering provider-driven care to delivering augmented care. In the both scenario (D4), VCT centers grow at 10 percent per year while augmented care crowds out ordinary public treatment facilities at 20 percent per year.[2]

## Effects of Alternative ART Policies

Projections of the effect of the VCT or the augmented policy on the future trajectory of the epidemic amount to careful calculations of the consequences of the assumptions presented in chapter 3 regarding the average effect on an individual's disease progression of either early recruitment or NGO support. Figure 5.1 displays

**Table 5.2** Policy Assumptions for the VCT, Augmented, and Both Scenarios

| | Scenario | | |
|---|---|---|---|
| *Parameter* | *VCT (D2)* | *Augmented (D3)* | *Both (D4)* |
| 1. Price of VCT (baht) | 30 | 30 | 30 |
| 2. Weight of short-run VCT demand in total (%) | 100.0 | 100.0 | 100.0 |
| 3. Growth rate of VCT facilities (%) | 15.0 | 0.0 | 10.0 |
| *Prices of ART (baht)* | | | |
| 4. Public | 650 | 650 | 650 |
| 5. Augmented public | 1,880 | 650 | 650 |
| 6. Private | 9,534 | 9,534 | 9,534 |
| 7. No ART | 30 | 30 | 30 |
| *Quantities of ART in 2003 (number of facilities)* | | | |
| 8. Public | 860 | 860 | 860 |
| 9. Augmented public | 100 | 100 | 100 |
| 10. Private | 100 | 100 | 100 |
| 11. No ART (residual) | 10,282 | 10,282 | 10,282 |
| *Other ART supply parameters* | | | |
| 12. Growth rate of ART facilities (%) | 2.5 | 1.5 | 2.5 |
| 13. Growth rate of augmented ART facilities (%) | 5.0 | 20.0 | 20.0 |
| 14. Growth rate of private ART facilities (%) | 4.0 | 2.0 | 3.0 |
| 15. Starting number of treatment slots per public facility (average) | 54 | 54 | 54 |
| 16. Starting number of treatment slots per augmented public facility (average) | 56 | 56 | 56 |
| 17. Proportion of treatment capacity designated to symptomatic patients before asymptomatic patients with CD4 < 200 cells/mm$^3$ are accepted (%) | 90.0 | 90.0 | 90.0 |
| 18. Growth rate of all public health facilities | 2.0 | 2.0 | 2.0 |
| 19. Number of treatment slots in 2002 | 8,341 | 8,341 | 8,341 |
| 20. Number of treatment slots in 2003 | 16,663 | 16,663 | 16,663 |

*Source:* MOPH data and authors' estimates.

the projected consequences of these policies in relation to the basic NAPHA policy. All three enhancement policies substantially increase the number of people living with HIV/AIDS (PHAs). The augmented policy without early recruitment is estimated to be about three times as effective in this regard as the early recruitment policy. But adding early recruitment (D2) to augmentation (D3) adds an additional 10,000 people to the ranks of people surviving with HIV/AIDS in 2025.[3]

Figure 5.2 shows that all three alternative policies postpone deaths that would have occurred under the NAPHA policy. Again, the aug-

**Figure 5.1** Projected Current HIV Cases under Alternative Scenarios Relative to NAPHA

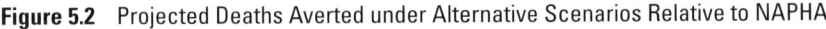

*Source:* Authors.
*Note:* Scenario D2 = VCT policy; scenario D3 = augmented public policy; scenario D4 = both
(VCT + augmented) policy.

**Figure 5.2** Projected Deaths Averted under Alternative Scenarios Relative to NAPHA

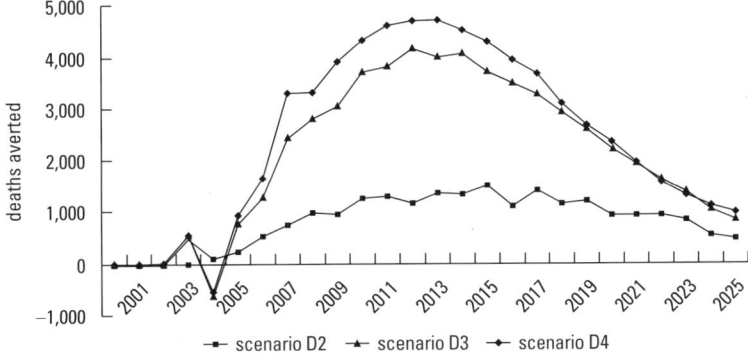

*Source:* Authors.
*Note:* Scenario D2 = VCT policy; scenario D3 = augmented public policy; scenario D4 = both
(VCT + augmented) policy.

mented policy (D3) is superior to the VCT policy (D2), and the both
policy (D4) dominates the other two. In 2010, for example, the
NAPHA policy would avert about 15,000 deaths in comparison with
the baseline. Figure 5.2 shows that in 2010 the both policy (D4) would
avert an additional 4,400 deaths, an improvement of about 30 percent.

These social (and private) gains are the result of keeping more people on ART. Figure 5.3 shows how many additional people will be on
ART in each year in comparison with the NAPHA scenario. The
ranking is the same, with the augmented scenario (D3) keeping about
60,000 additional people on ART, more than twice as many as would

**Figure 5.3** Projected HIV-Positive People on ART under Alternative Scenarios Relative to NAPHA

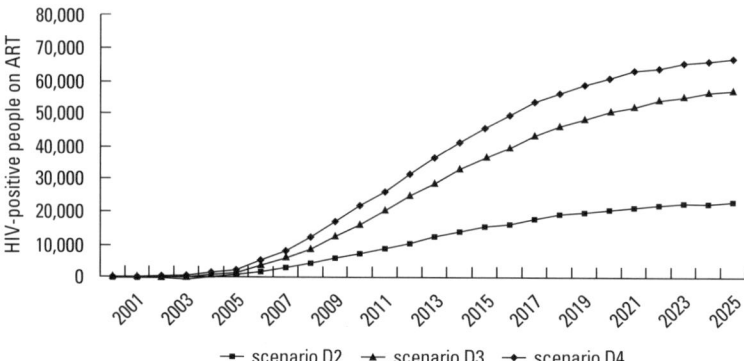

*Source:* Authors.
*Note:* Scenario D2 = VCT policy; scenario D3 = augmented public policy; scenario D4 = both (VCT + augmented) policy.

**Figure 5.4** Projected Annual Life-Years Saved under Alternative Scenarios Relative to NAPHA

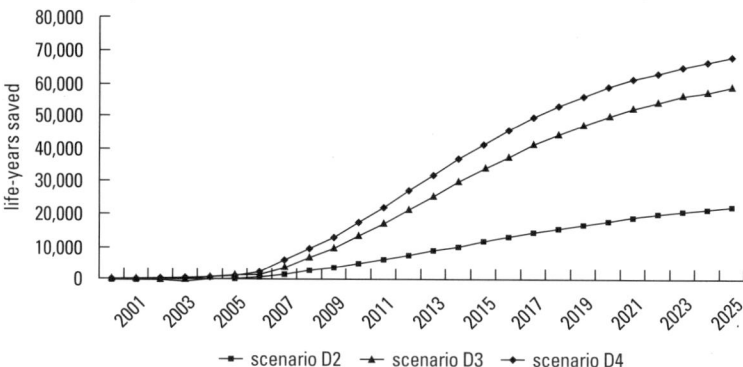

*Source:* Authors.
*Note:* Scenario D2 = VCT policy; scenario D3 = augmented public policy; scenario D4 = both (VCT + augmented) policy.

be added in the VCT scenario (D2). Again, the both scenario (D4) accumulates the largest number of ART patients.

The result of these enhancement policies is to increase the number of life-years saved in each year. These incremental benefits are shown in figure 5.4 to be quite high. We showed in chapter 4 that by starting people on ART in 2002 (the NAPHA scenario) about 210,000 more people would be alive in 2020. Figure 5.2 shows that the VCT, augmented, and both policies save (respectively) 18,000, 50,000, and

60,000 additional life-years in that year. Thus, the alternative policies offer the possibility of improving the benefits in 2020 by almost 30 percent.

These projections tell us the incremental benefits of the enhanced policies. Now we turn to consideration of their incremental costs.

## Costs of Alternative ART Policies

Figure 5.5 shows the projections of the net cost of the NAPHA policy and of the three enhanced policies. The *net cost* is defined as the total cost of ART plus the cost of any VCT expenses, minus the cost of any reduced expenditure on the treatment of opportunistic infections. The bottom line in the figure gives the projection of the net cost of the NAPHA scenario, which is very similar to the projected gross cost of NAPHA (D1) given in figure 4.14. The two estimates are similar because VCT costs are small in the NAPHA policy and savings from reduced opportunistic infections are small relative to the magnitude of ART costs.

According to these projections, the VCT (D2) and the augmented (D3) policies have roughly similar costs, while the both (D4) policy is about 10 percent more costly than either. Even the most expensive of the policies never exceeds 30 percent of the projected national health budget, which itself is only 1.3 percent of the entire national budget.[4]

**Figure 5.5** Projected Net Cost of ART for All Four Scenarios

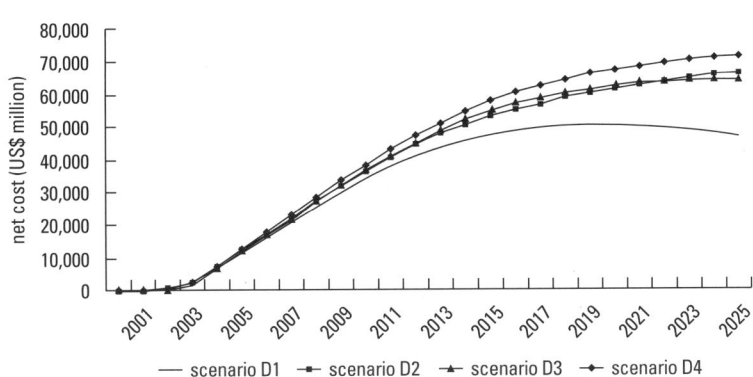

*Source:* Authors.
*Note:* Scenario D1 = NAPHA policy; scenario D2 = VCT policy; scenario D3 = augmented public policy; scenario D4 = both (VCT + augmented) policy.

## The Cost-Effectiveness of Alternative ART Policy Scenarios

Assembling the costs and effects of the four policies allows two types of analysis. First, one can analyze the cost-effectiveness of any of the four against the baseline. At this early stage in Thailand's implementation of NAPHA, such an analysis can guide current policy into a more cost-effective path. One can instead consider the NAPHA scenario (D1) as a new point of comparison and analyze the cost-effectiveness of the VCT (D2), augmented (D3), or both (D4) policy in comparison with that new baseline. The advantage of this approach is that, where an enhanced policy costs more per life-year saved, one can ask whether the additional life-years saved are worth the extra expenditure.

Figure 5.6 presents the first of these analyses. Of the four policies, the current baseline NAPHA policy (D1) is the most cost-effective. The second most cost-effective is the augmented policy (D3). This finding is not surprising because the augmented policy achieves two or three times as many incremental life-years saved at roughly the same cost as the VCT scenario (D2). Because it combines the two "pure" enhancement strategies, the cost per year of the both scenario (D4) lies between the costs per year of the other two scenarios.

If all four policies achieved the same objectives, it would be wise to choose the most cost-effective, eschewing the enhancements. However, we have already seen that the enhanced policies achieve more than the simple NAPHA policy. Each enhancement saves additional life-years at some additional cost. In comparison with the NAPHA

**Figure 5.6** Cost-Effectiveness of NAPHA and Alternative Scenarios Relative to Baseline

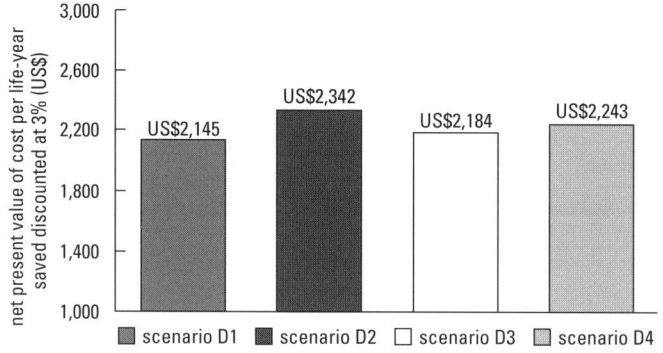

*Source:* Authors.
*Note:* Scenario D1 = NAPHA policy; scenario D2 = VCT policy; scenario D3 = augmented public policy; scenario D4 = both (VCT + augmented) policy.

scenario, the projections predict that the VCT scenario would save an additional 144,737 discounted life-years, whereas the augmented scenario would save an additional 414,840 life-years. Implementing both enhancements would save 490,844 life-years in addition to those saved by the NAPHA baseline policy.

The decision on whether to enhance NAPHA in any of these three ways should be based on the costs of these additional health benefits. The cost projections predict that the present value of the additional expenditures required to save the 144,737 life-years would be US$860 million (B 33.6 billion), or about US$5,941 (B 237,640) for every additional life-year for the VCT scenario. Because the augmented scenario is projected to cost an additional US$1 billion (discounted dollars), (B 40 billion) it could be used to add to the health benefits at a cost of US$2,430 (B 97,200) per additional life-year saved. The program combining both of these two enhancements would cost an additional US$1.3 billion (B 52 billion), or an average of US$2,77 (B 110,840) per additional life-year saved. These costs are displayed in figure 5.7.

In view of those results, which program should Thailand undertake? The answer depends on the value that Thailand places on a life-year saved. Suppose that value is US$2,200 (B 88,000). This number is greater than the cost per life-year saved under NAPHA but less than the incremental cost per life-year saved under any of the three enhanced programs. In this case, assuming that Thailand has already exhausted all other opportunities to save years of life for less than US$2,200 (B 88,000), the country should choose the basic NAPHA modeled here.

**Figure 5.7**  Cost-Effectiveness of Alternative Scenarios Relative to NAPHA

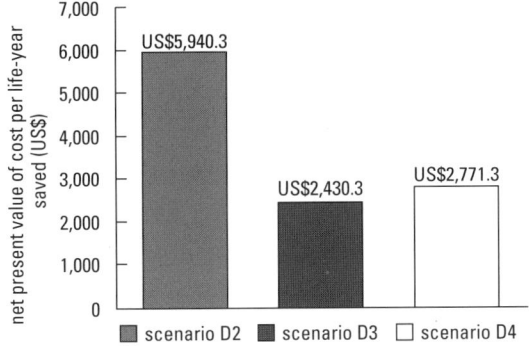

*Source:* Authors.
*Note:* D2 = VCT policy; scenario D3 = augmented public policy; scenario D4 = both (VCT + augmented) policy.

It should leave the enhancements to the private decisions of individuals who are able to appreciate them and are willing to pay for their incremental costs out of their own pockets or from health insurance.

Suppose instead that Thailand attaches a value of US$4,000 (B 160,000), or about twice its gross national income per capita, to the life-year saved. Because some international experts suggest that a life-year could be valued as high as five times the per capita income, a valuation of US$4,000 (B 160,000) would not be extremely high for Thailand. In that case, Thailand should aspire to achieve the maximum health benefits suggested by this analysis, which are attainable only through the most generous program. The cost-effectiveness of enhancing the basic program with both (a) VCT and (b) PHA and NGO demand-side augmentation is quite attractive, at only US$2,771 (B 110,840) per additional life-year saved.

Regardless of the value that Thailand places on life-years, this analysis suggests that the country should not adopt a policy that improves only VCT recruitment without improving adherence. That scenario, labeled D2 in figure 5.7, is clearly dominated by the other two enhanced policies.

## Fiscal and Financial Implications of ART Policy Scenarios

In chapter 4, we compared the projected annual flow of expenditures on public ART with the projected levels of the AIDS and health budgets through 2025. This section adds a similar analysis of the enhanced scenarios. It also compares the projected public expenditure per life-year to the incomes of the various income groups in Thailand, in order to assess the private affordability of treatment.

### Compare All Four Scenarios with AIDS Budget

Figure 5.8 shows that the major budget implications of choosing one of the enhanced scenarios will not be felt until the outer years of the projection period, when the both scenario (D4) will cost about one-fourth more than the basic NAPHA scenario (D1). The figure also shows how these costs compare with a projection of the recent AIDS budget, which is assumed to grow at only the projected growth rate of gross domestic product—5.2 percent. Panel (a) of figure 5.8 indicates

**Figure 5.8** ART Cost of NAPHA and Alternative ART Scenarios

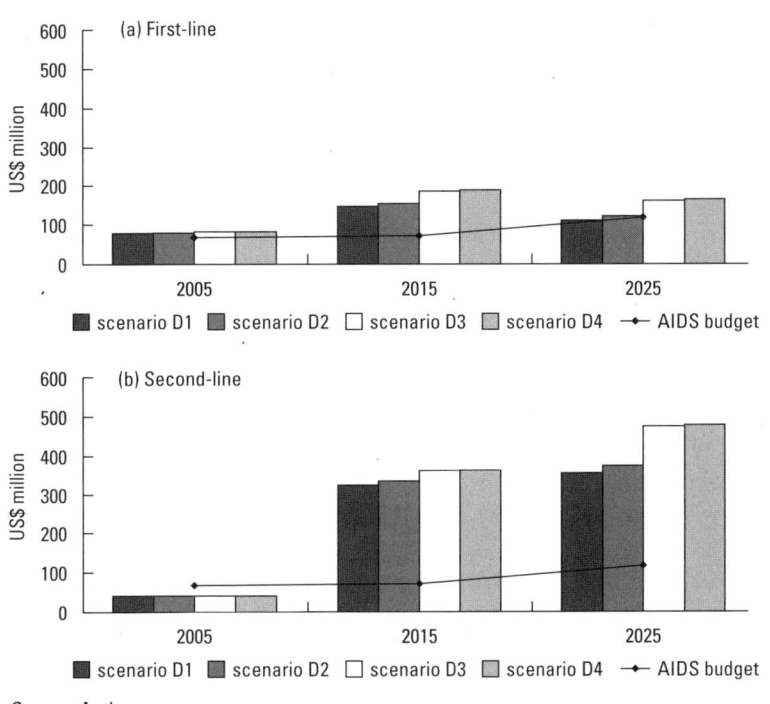

*Source:* Authors.
*Note:* Scenario D2 = VCT policy; scenario D3 = augmented public policy; scenario D4 = both (VCT + augmented) policy.

that, unless the AIDS budget grows faster than gross domestic product, the cost of first-line ART can easily exhaust the AIDS budget; however, panel (b) shows that second-line therapy will have a substantially larger budget impact. Already by 2015 the projected cost of the second-line therapy alone will be more than three times greater than the projected level of recent AIDS budgets.

As discussed earlier, recent AIDS or health sector budgets provide no sure way of judging the affordability of any project. Suppose Thailand has the opportunity to invest in life-saving therapy at a cost of US$2,430 (B 97,200) per life-year and has exhausted other opportunities to lengthen the productive lifetimes of its citizens at this cost. Its decision on whether to spend this money should be based not on any putative criterion of affordability but simply on whether it values healthy life-years at least this highly. If it does, then it should either tax or borrow to finance these expenditures.

## *Affordability to Private Households*

An alternative to public financing for ART would be to finance all or part of its cost through user fees. Table 5.3 shows the private afford-ability of ART by household income level. According to the socioeco-nomic survey data for 2002, the mean nominal income per household for the poorest 20 percent was US$4,043 (B 161,720), of which US$1,678 (B 67,120) was spent on nonfood expenditure and US$300 (B 12,000) on medical expenditure in an average year. The highest income quintile, in contrast, has about 10 times more income and spends about 12 times more on medical expenses in the average year.

Comparing the cost of ART with these household averages is diffi-cult. First, households with AIDS patients might have been different from households without such patients—either poorer or richer—even before the AIDS patient became sick.[5] Second, the sickness is likely to reduce the productivity of the patient and therefore the

**Table 5.3**  Affordability of First- and Second-Line ART by Household Income

| | Quintile | | | | |
|---|---|---|---|---|---|
| | 1 (poorest) | Q2 | Q3 | Q4 | 5 (richest) |
| Mean household income (US$) | 4,042.70 | 6,678.10 | 9,806.10 | 15,434.00 | 40,253.20 |
| Nonfood expenditure, household (US$) | 1,678.40 | 3,127.90 | 4,983.90 | 8,525.30 | 25,597.60 |
| Medical expenditure, household (US$) | 300.00 | 512.30 | 754.70 | 1,165.50 | 3,633.00 |
| Cost of ART (first-line) | 842.20 | 842.20 | 842.20 | 842.20 | 842.20 |
| Cost of ART (second-line) | 6,960.20 | 6,960.20 | 6,960.20 | 6,960.20 | 6,960.20 |
| Cost of ART (first-line) as | | | | | |
| Share of household income (%) | 21 | 13 | 9 | 5 | 2 |
| Share of nonfood expenditure (%) | 50 | 27 | 17 | 10 | 3 |
| Share of medical expenditure (%) | 281 | 164 | 112 | 72 | 23 |
| Cost of ART (second-line) as | | | | | |
| Share of household income (%) | 172 | 104 | 71 | 45 | 17 |
| Share of nonfood expenditure (%) | 415 | 223 | 140 | 82 | 27 |
| Share of medical expenditure (%) | 2,320 | 1,359 | 922 | 597 | 192 |

*Source:* Authors' calculations based on Thailand socioeconomic survey in 2002.
*Note:* All monetary amounts are in 2004 U.S. dollars.

income of the household. Third, household membership itself is flexible: households can recruit new members to help care for a sick person or can seek temporary alternative homes for household members who need to be free of the burden of the sickness. The AIDS patient may move to a new household, perhaps to be closer to a treatment site or a valued caregiver.

Setting aside these concerns, we note that the annual cost of first-line ART is substantially greater than average annual medical expenditures only in the poorest 40 percent of the households. Accordingly, for the top half of the households in the income distribution, first-line ART is affordable. Even for the poorest half of the households, the US$842 (B 33,680) cost of first-line therapy compares with the medical expenses of the sickest households for a single year.

The problems for the poorest households are likely to be caused by two unusual features of the cost of treatment:

• The treatment must continue for the rest of the patient's life. For households in the lowest 80 percent of the income distribution that might be able to raise the resources to pay US$842 (B 33,680) for one year, payment for the second and third year will become onerous.

• Laxity in treatment will lead to treatment failure, the development of resistant strains of the virus, the spread of those resistant strains to others, and the requirement that the patient move to second-line therapy. All these repercussions are extremely negative for the patient and, in the case of the transmitted resistant strain of the virus, for society.

To the extent that a higher price for first-line therapy leads to a higher failure rate for first-line therapy, it increases the costs of AIDS to the individual and to society.

The option of cofinancing ART with user fees deserves fuller treatment than is possible here. However, we stress that any price-induced reduction in adherence will have negative spillover effects. Comparison of first-line costs with household income and expenditure levels (in figure 5.9) suggests that even first-line therapy is difficult for the poorest households to finance, especially over the longer run. Careful attention should be given to determining which patients will

**Figure 5.9** Affordability of ART by Income Level

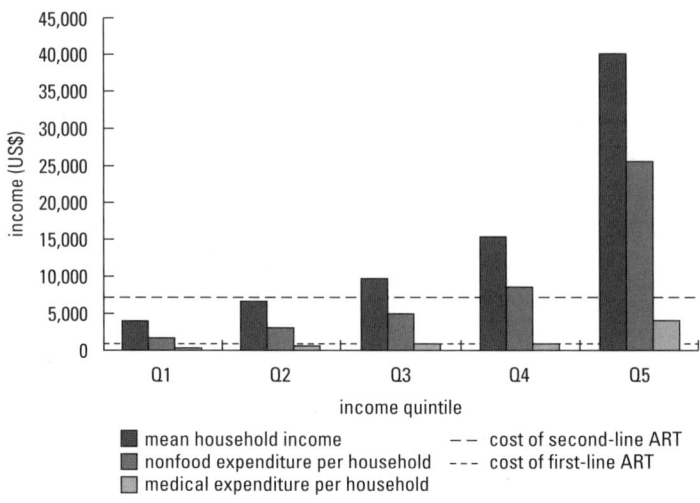

*Source:* Authors.

adhere—despite paying a higher price—and which will not. Those who will not should receive free care—or should even be rewarded for good adherence. In other words, perhaps the price to some patients should be negative.

Although the cost of first-line therapy could be partially financed with user fees, second-line therapy is much more expensive, exceeding total household income for 40 percent of the population. A large proportion of those on first-line therapy will eventually need second-line therapy. Furthermore, poor adherence to first-line therapy speeds the development of resistance to those drugs and hastens the day when the patient must move to second-line therapy. Accordingly, from a social as well as an individual perspective, adherence support mechanisms such as the augmented public care we model in this report are likely to be cost-effective as well as therapeutically beneficial.

Given the potentially important contribution that NGO or PHA support groups might make to adherence, if they effectively augment public (and perhaps also private) care, the problem of financing should perhaps be posed as one of designing the optimal financing mechanism for these groups. If membership dues increase the stability and the accountability of these groups to their constituents, then perhaps this form of user fee should be explored in addition to—or instead of—fees paid directly to the health care system.

## NAPHA Policy without Brand-Name Second-Line Pharmaceutical Products

In chapter 4, financial analysis of the NAPHA policy demonstrated that second-line drug costs account for most of the annual budget after a few years, though only a minority of patients use them. However, virtually all patients eventually need second-line therapy. Hence, excluding second-line drugs from NAPHA reduces the health benefits of the program and shortens the life expectancy of patients. Despite growing needs and demands from the PHA and international AIDS communities, at present the Thai government has not yet made an explicit decision regarding public provision of ART, beyond the currently available drug regimens for first-line therapy. In this section, we compare the benefits and costs of the basic NAPHA policy analyzed in chapter 4 with a version of the policy that excludes second-line therapy. We assume the resulting cost savings are absorbed entirely by the government, leaving no cost implications for the patient from this change. Consequently, the demand for VCT and for treatment does not change relative to our earlier scenarios.

### Projected Costs

Figure 5.10 presents the projected cost of the NAPHA scenario with and without second-line therapy. The cost of NAPHA with second-line therapy is reproduced from figure 4.14. With second-line drugs, NAPHA costs increase sharply to an inflection point in 2008–09 and then level off to a ceiling of US$500 million (B 20 billion) by 2017. In contrast, the

**Figure 5.10** Projected ART Costs of NAPHA Scenarios with and without Second-Line ART

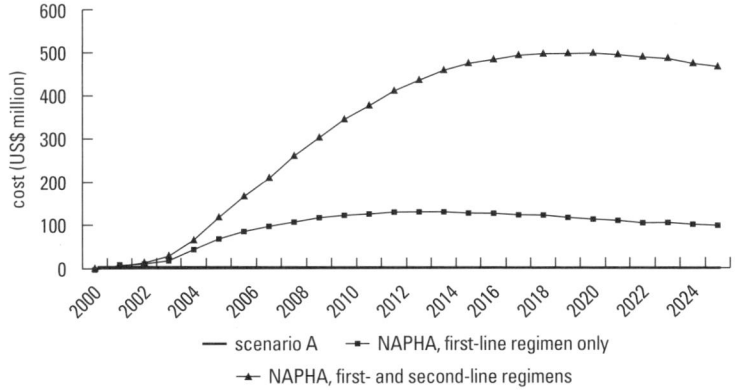

- scenario A    NAPHA, first-line regimen only
    NAPHA, first- and second-line regimens

*Source:* Authors.

**Figure 5.11**  Projected Annual Costs and Benefits of NAPHA Scenario without Second-Line ART

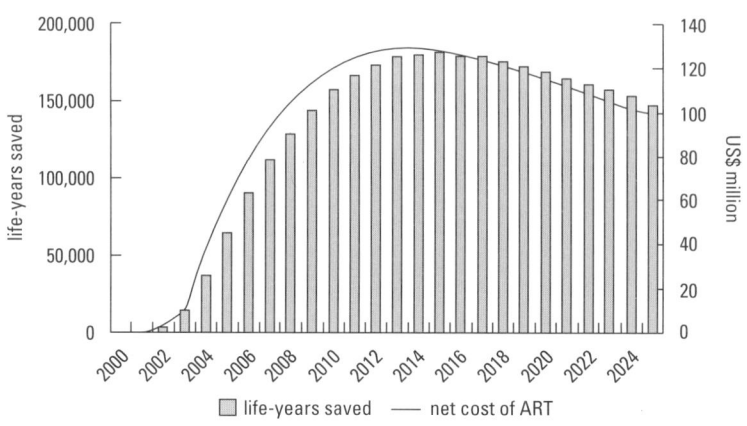

Source: Authors.

NAPHA policy using only first-line drugs costs only about one-fifth as much as it would when second-line drugs are included. When second-line drugs are not included, the total cost peaks at about US$130 million (B 5.2 billion) per year in 2013, before leveling off.

### Projected Costs and Benefits

Excluding coverage for second-line drugs (and assuming patients do not buy them on their own) reduces the benefits of NAPHA as well as the costs. Figure 5.11 presents both the benefits (on the left vertical axis) and the costs (on the right vertical axis) of NAPHA without second-line drugs. In comparison with the similar figure 4.17, the line graph representing health benefits rises almost as high but declines more quickly, with only about 150,000 survivors in 2025 instead of the almost 200,000 survivors when second-line drugs are included. In contrast, the costs to the government remain about US$120 million (B 4,800) per year, or about one-fifth the value when second-line drugs are included.

### Cost-Effectiveness Analysis

Figure 5.12 presents the cost per life-year saved of NAPHA without second-line therapy compared with the cost per life-year saved of NAPHA with second-line therapy (from chapter 4). The central finding is that NAPHA can save a year of life for US$2,145 (B 85,800).[6] The figure shows that NAPHA with first-line therapy only, at just

**Figure 5.12** Cost-Effectiveness of NAPHA Scenarios with and without Second-Line ART

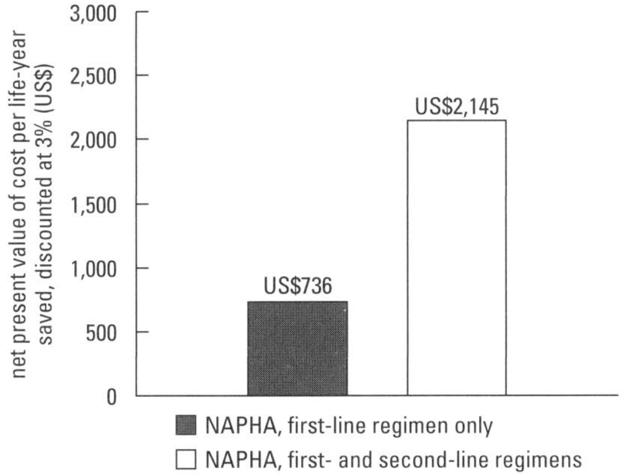

*Source:* Authors.

US$736 (B 29,440) per discounted life-year saved, is far more cost-effective than NAPHA with second-line therapy, which costs US$2,145 (B 85,800) per discounted life-year saved. (As before, a discount rate of 3 percent per year was used to compute the net present values of the future streams of costs and benefits.)

This result poses important questions for the Royal Thai government: Should it commit to public provision of the much more expensive second-line therapy in addition to first-line therapy? Or should it limit its commitment to providing only first-line therapy, with a promise to provide palliative care for those who fail first-line treatment? In the absence of significant change in the price of second-line drugs, the cost of saving an additional life-year through second-line therapy is high when compared with the substantial health benefits of first-line policy only. On a pure cost-effectiveness basis, a policy with first-line therapy only would be superior.[7]

## Notes

1.  The discussion of figure 4.8 presents the methods used to project the effect of improved VCT accessibility on the use of VCT.

2.  The transformation of hundreds of public treatment locations into augmented public treatment locations would make it difficult to grow the VCT centers at 15 percent per year. So we decrease that target to 10 percent a year in this scenario.

3. As noted in chapter 4, these projections assume that the choice of treatment policy does not affect risk behavior. Consequently, these additional HIV-infected people are the result of improved survival and the fact that longer-lived HIV-infected people have more opportunity to transmit infections.

4. The cost projections in this study do not attach a shadow price to the cost of public sector resources. Because such shadow prices are typically about 10 percent, these projections could be understating the opportunity costs of AIDS programs by roughly 10 percent.

5. For example, in Kagera, Tanzania, households that experienced the death of a prime-age adult tended to be wealthier before the death than were other households (World Bank 1999).

6. The two cost-effectiveness estimates for Thailand reported in figure 5.12 are both greater than was estimated by a similar study of India, which concluded that ART would improve health at a cost of less than US$300 (B 12,000) per life-year in that country (Over and others 2004). The difference in costs is due partly to the higher clinical costs estimated for Thailand and, in the case of the US$2,145 figure (B 85,800), to the inclusion of second-line therapy, which was excluded from consideration in the India study.

7. If NAPHA without first-line therapy is taken as the base case, then the addition of second-line therapy will save a further 395,665 discounted life-years at an additional cost of nearly US$4 billion (B 160 billion) over a projected 23 years. Hence, the cost of the additional life-year gained by adding second-line therapy will be approximately US$10,000 (B 400,000) per life year. This is a great deal of money at Thailand's level of gross national income, especially in comparison with the US$736 (B 29,440) that the government would be paying for the substantial health benefits of the first-line-only NAPHA policy. Whether the government decides to finance second-line therapy depends on whether political constituencies support the free provision of second-line therapy and also on whether second-line drugs can be obtained at prices much lower than current prices.

# CHAPTER 6

# Sensitivity of the Policy Rankings
# to Key Assumptions

The preceding chapters construct a model of the economics and epidemiology of antiretroviral therapy (ART) in order to arrive at concrete estimates of the cost-effectiveness of the NAPHA (National Access to Antiretrovirals Program for People Living with AIDS) policy and of three alternative enhancements to it. The empirical support for the many assumptions behind the model varies from substantial for some assumptions—such as the survival patterns for people with HIV/AIDS who do not receive treatment—to weak for others—such as the responsiveness of the demand for voluntary counseling and testing (VCT) to price and distance by risk group. Other assumptions pertain to the evolution of technology and prices, matters on which we can only make informed guesses.

One approach to the existing uncertainty on all these matters is to make policy by instinct, without reference to any explicit model. Frequently policy makers are forced to enact policy in exactly this way. However, to the extent that policies have any logic, they are based on an implicit model and its assumptions. Because they are not explicitly discussed, these implicit models may contain internal inconsistencies or depend critically on unstated assumptions. They may therefore lead policy makers and their constituents into making mistakes that could have been avoided using an explicit model.

The advantage of using an explicit model, as we have done here, is that the assumptions can be made explicit and their influence on the results can be studied using sensitivity analysis.

## Sensitivity to Alternative Biological and Price Assumptions

In this chapter, we perform sensitivity analysis for two groups of assumptions:

• First, we study the effect of alternative assumptions regarding key biological features of antiretroviral medicine and the prices at which ART drugs can be purchased.

• Second, we analyze the effects of alternative behavioral assumptions.

All analyses are performed in comparison with the projections of NAPHA including second-line therapy that are presented in chapter 4.

### *Key Biological Parameters*

Several biological assumptions affect the results. We report sensitivity analysis regarding two: infectivity and resistance.

#### *Infectivity*
In our baseline model, we assume that the infectivity of people on ART is reduced by 75 percent. To measure the sensitivity of the results to this assumption, we run both optimistic and pessimistic scenarios (100 percent reduction versus no reduction). Figure 6.1 reports the effect of the infectivity assumption on a key indicator of epidemic growth: the number of new HIV infections in any given year. The central curve, which peaks at 1,823 in 2012 and then declines asymptotically to 1,000, presents the number of additional new HIV infections transmitted under NAPHA by the people who remain healthy because of ART. Because the trend toward safer behavior is assumed to be unchanged by ART, these additional HIV infections are caused solely by the increased longevity of AIDS patients.

The baseline projection in the absence of NAPHA (scenario A1) predicts that the number of new HIV infections would decline from 17,000 in 2003 to about 3,600 in 2015 and then to about 2,400 in 2025. In comparison with these baseline numbers, the central curve in figure 6.1 shows that NAPHA will substantially increase the number of new infections, especially in the later years. In percentage terms, NAPHA increases the number of new HIV infections by about 40 percent in each year between 2012 through 2025. The bottom curve

**Figure 6.1** New HIV Cases by Infectivity Rates among People on ART: NAPHA Scenario

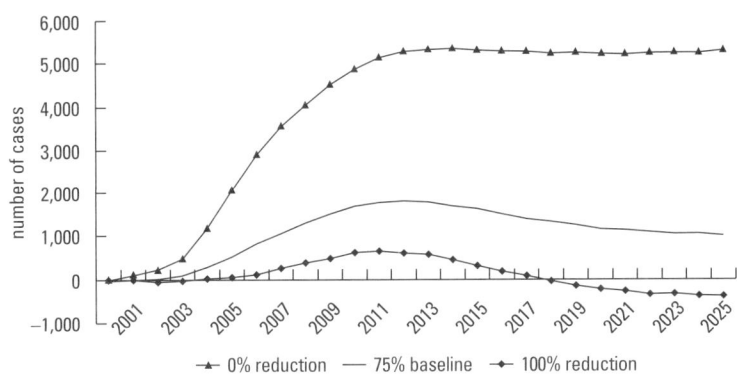

*Source:* Authors.

in figure 6.1 shows that the number of new infections is reduced if ART is assumed to completely eliminate transmission by the infected person (100 percent reduction). In this case, the only increase in new infections attributable to NAPHA is the result of treatment failure, when ART can no longer sustain health or impede transmission.

The top curve in figure 6.1 shows that the spillover effect from greater longevity would be far greater if, as argued by Auvert and others (2004), ART had no biological impact on infectivity. By increasing the number of new infections by about 5,000 in every year after 2011, NAPHA would more than double the new infections in every year after 2012 and would triple the number of new infections in the last four years of the projection, from about 2,500 per year to about 7,500 per year.

Despite its sizable effect on the number of new HIV cases, a change in the infectivity rate has a relatively minor effect on the cost-effectiveness results, as shown in figure 6.2. Under the worst-case scenario of zero reduction in infectivity for ART patients, the cost per life-year saved of NAPHA rises by only 5 percent, from US$2,145 (B 85,800) for the basic program to US$2,257 (B 90,280). This result follows directly from our adoption of a finite planning horizon of 2025. Because progression from HIV infection to a need for treatment takes a median time of seven years and first-line therapy will sustain people from that point for several more years, few of those infected by AIDS patients in any of these scenarios will progress to expensive second-line therapy before the end of the planning period.

**Figure 6.2**  Net Present Value of Cost per Life-Year Saved by Infectivity Scenario

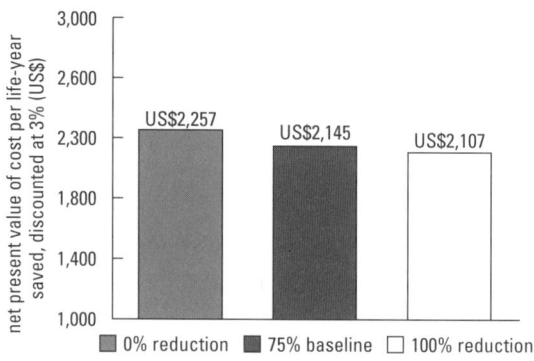

*Source:* Authors.

*Resistance*

The second key assumption used in the analysis is a rate of resistance among the ART patients for whom first-line ART therapy failed. The model uses the assumption that 80 percent of people on ART develop resistance strains when first-line ART therapy fails for them. In Thailand, we assume that because of the lack of physicians experienced with ART treatment and the limited availability of viral-load testing at district level facilities, some 20 percent of ART patients are switched to second-line ART without having any resistant strains. However, more trained physicians and wider availability of viral-load testing throughout the country would reduce this proportion and allow only patients with resistant virus to switch to second-line ART therapy.

We conducted sensitivity analysis by using resistance assumptions of 50 and 100 percent. The results indicate that with 100 percent resistance approximately 23 percent more HIV-positive people carry resistant strains by 2025 than do under our starting assumption of 80 percent resistance. When a 50 percent resistance rate is used instead, the prevalence of resistant strains is reduced by 14 percent. However, again because of the 20-year planning horizon, these changes make almost no difference in the number of new HIV cases or the cost per life-year saved.

### Price of First- and Second-Line ART Therapy

Chapter 3 presented the estimated unit cost for both first- and second-line therapy based on current drug regimens and using the current prices of both generic and branded drugs in Thailand. If current efforts by multinational pharmaceutical manufacturers to extend patent protection to second-line drugs are successful, the prices of second-line drugs are likely to remain high. However, if such efforts fail, the prices of second-line drugs could fall by as much as we have seen the prices of first-line drugs decline in recent years. However, recent legislative changes in India to comply with the World Trade Organization's Agreement on Trade-Related Aspects of Intellectual Property Rights (TRIPS)[1] raise concern that the costs of the raw materials that Thailand imports from India to make its GPO-vir will rise in price, forcing cost increases in GPO-vir, which is used in first-line therapy.

In this section, we keep the technical specification of ART unchanged (for second- as well as first-line therapy) in order to compute the cost-effectiveness of the following:

• 50 percent reduction in the price of second-line ART therapy

• 25 percent reduction in the price of first-line therapy and a 50 percent reduction in the price of second-line therapy

• 25 percent increase in the price of first-line therapy.

In all simulations, we assume that the price to the patient remains unchanged, so that patient behavior does not change and the government absorbs all the cost savings from the reduction.[2]

The results of these alternative price assumptions regarding the prices of first- and second-line therapies are displayed in the four panels of figure 6.3. Panel (a) repeats the findings of chapter 5, which showed that NAPHA is the most cost-effective option, followed by augmented care. The other three panels present the cost-effectiveness results of varying the first- and second-line drug prices as specified above.

Panels (b) and (c) show that if the price of second-line therapy were reduced by 50 percent, the cost-effectiveness of all policy scenarios would greatly improve. Unlike the "no second-line" option simulated at the end of chapter 5, these simulations retain the health benefits of second-line therapy but pay less for them. They suggest the potential benefits to Thailand of negotiating much better prices on second-line drugs from multinational corporations or, alternatively, of compulsory licensing of these pharmaceuticals.

**Figure 6.3** Sensitivity of the Cost-Effectiveness Analysis to Prices of First- and Second-Line ART

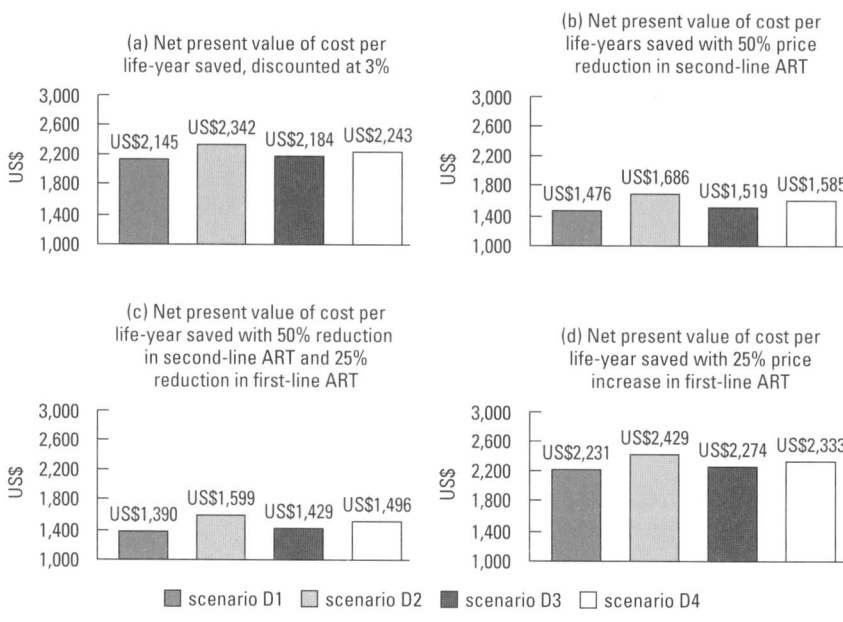

Source: Authors.

Panel (d) shows the result of higher prices for first-line therapy (perhaps caused by the new legislation in India) with unchanged prices for second-line therapy. This set of simulations shows that in a context where many people receive expensive second-line care, a small increase in the cost of first-line drugs could be absorbed relatively easily. However, if second-line drugs were unavailable, the same increase in the cost of first-line drugs would be larger in percentage terms and might cause a political reaction.

In none of the four panels does the ranking of policy options change. In all four, the pure NAPHA policy (scenario D1) remains the most cost-effective. In all four, the increase in cost per life-year saved of the both option (scenario D4) over the NAPHA-only option is small, given that the both option saves many more lives. Accordingly, in all four cases the recommendation would be to choose the both scenario, which enhances public ART delivery with both early recruitment (using VCT) and adherence support (using groups of people living with HIV/AIDS).[3]

## Sensitivity to Changes in Risk Behavior

The simulation modeling performed in chapters 4 and 5 assumes that treatment policy does not affect risk behavior. This assumption may not be the case. As pointed out in chapter 2 and in the bottom row of table 3.8 in chapter 3, risk behavior may respond either positively or negatively to the availability of effective low-cost ART. We model a positive effect of ART availability on the demand for VCT (through responsiveness to lower price and distance to ART). However, in the basic policy and epidemiological models used in chapters 4 and 5, we permit no direct effect of VCT on risk behavior. In the baseline scenario and in the four policy scenarios, risk behavior continues to improve gradually following the trend of the past 15 years, when ART was neither very effective nor easily available. This section presents the results of sensitivity analysis with respect to risk behavior. Using the NAPHA policy (scenario D1) from chapter 4 as the benchmark, this section shows how the cost per life-year saved would be affected by either "beneficial" or "adverse" behavioral reactions of different groups of the population.

Table 6.1 presents the alternative assumptions about risk behavior for which sensitivity analysis is performed. The first column of the table presents the central assumptions under which all of the simulations of scenarios A, D1, D2, D3, and D4 are computed in chapters 4 and 5. The second and third data columns present, respectively, the beneficial assumptions and the adverse assumptions regarding behavioral response to treatment availability.

The sensitivity analysis compares the NAPHA cost-effectiveness result under the unchanged central behavioral assumptions—US$2,145 (B 85,800) per life-year saved—with the cost-effectiveness of NAPHA when behavior changes in response to treatment. Four types of behavioral response are considered:

- baseline behavior using central assumptions
- beneficial
- adverse
- extremely adverse

A beneficial behavioral response associates improved treatment availability with improved condom use in all risk groups. Condom use is assumed to increase from the central assumptions used in all previous scenarios to the beneficial assumptions listed in table 6.1. The result: the number of life-years saved is greater at the same or lower treatment cost. Cost-effectiveness is improved. According to the simulations, the results of which are depicted in figure 6.4, the cost per life-year saved drops from US$2,145 to US$1,952, an improvement of about 9 percent.

An adverse behavioral response is simulated by assuming that condom use in all risk groups declines from the central levels previously assumed to the lower levels presented in the "adverse" column of table 6.1. In this case, as figure 6.4 shows, the cost-effectiveness of the NAPHA policy deteriorates, from US$2,145 to US$2,487 (B 85,800 to B 99,480) per life-year saved.

We also simulated a mixed beneficial-adverse scenario by assuming that risk behavior among those on ART improves, while risk behavior among those not on ART deteriorates. The result of this combination of behavioral responses falls naturally between the adverse and beneficial results. However, since the groups whose behavior deteriorates are larger and include the major drivers of the epidemic, the result is closer to the adverse scenario than to the beneficial one. These results are omitted from the discussion and the figures.

Finally, we examined the behavior of the model under a set of extremely adverse assumptions. Here, we adopt the pessimistic

**Table 6.1** Proportion of Risky Sexual Acts Protected by Condoms: Alternative Behavioral Responses to Treatment Availability
*percentage*

| Risk groups | | Assumptions for behavioral change | | | |
|---|---|---|---|---|---|
| | | *Central* | *Beneficial* | *Adverse* | *Very adverse* |
| High | CSW | 85 | 95 | 75 | 60 |
| | Clients | 85 | 95 | 75 | 60 |
| | MSM | 85 | 95 | 75 | 60 |
| | IDU | 20 | 30 | 10 | 10 |
| Low | General male | 35 | 45 | 25 | 25 |
| | General female | 35 | 45 | 25 | 25 |
| **Risk groups** | | *Central* | *Beneficial* | *Adverse* | *Very adverse* |
| Percentage of men who visit | | | | | |
| Direct sex workers | | 10 | 5 | 20 | 20 |
| Indirect sex workers | | 10 | 5 | 20 | 20 |
| STI prevalence (among CSWs) | | 1.8 | 0.6 | 3.4 | 10.1 |

*Source:* Authors.
*Note:* CSW = commercial sex worker, MSM = men who have sex with men, IDU = injecting drug user, STI = sexually transmitted infection.

**Figure 6.4** Sensitivity of the Cost Effectiveness of NAPHA Policy to Risk Behavior

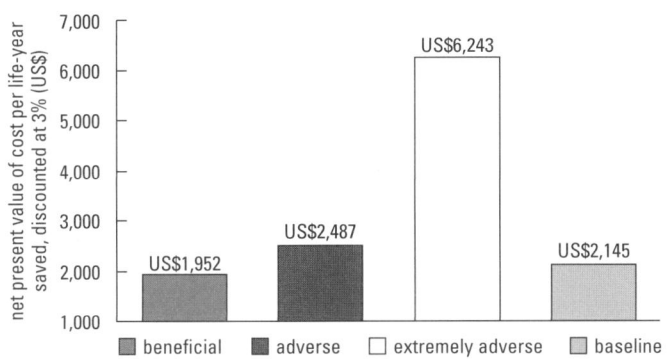

*Source:* Authors.
*Note:* Beneficial = beneficial effects (reduced risk behavior) of those who are on ART and those who are not on ART. Adverse = adverse effects (increased risk behavior) of those who are on ART and those who are not on ART. Extremely adverse = adverse effects (increased risk behavior) of those who are on ART and those who are not on ART, with the risk behavior at the same level as in 1980.

hypothesis that condom use in high-risk contacts, needle exchange among drug users, and the rates of prevalence of other sexually transmitted infections all return to levels not seen since the early to mid-1990s. In contrast to the "adverse" scenario described above, this "extremely adverse" scenario produces a dramatic acceleration in new HIV infections: 85,000 new infections per year by 2015, instead of only 5,000 under the NAPHA scenario with no change in risk behavior. By 2025, the annual number of new HIV infections rises to more than 180,000, as compared with less than 3,000 new infections under our baseline projection. Despite the 20-year planning horizon, which excludes most of the cost of treating these thousands of new infections, the cost per life-year saved for NAPHA would almost triple to US$6,243 (B 249,720).[4]

One lesson of this sensitivity analysis is that where effective prevention has already greatly limited the growth of the epidemic and condom use is quite high among almost all groups, the cost-effectiveness of ART is less sensitive to behavior than it would be in an epidemic like that in India, where infections are spreading rapidly from a core of high-risk populations into an unprotected general population. Nevertheless, the Thai government must guard against the possibility that extreme complacency would decrease condom use even more than we have assumed in our "adverse" scenario. Dramatic reductions in condom use would indeed reignite the epidemic. A second lesson from this section is that policies that use ART to effectively leverage improved prevention efforts might improve the cost-effectiveness of ART in Thailand by as much as 10 percent.

## Notes

1. Before 2005, Indian patent law differed from patent law elsewhere in granting patents exclusively on processes rather than on products. Under that law, Indian pharmaceutical manufacturers were able to legally produce copies of internationally patented drugs by developing novel processes for their production. To conform with World Trade Organization provisions on intellectual property rights, the Indian parliament passed a new Patents Act on March 23, 2005, which abolishes process patents in favor of product patents and recognizes international product patents. Under the new law, Indian pharmaceutical firms may be able to produce and sell internationally patented drugs, if those drugs were patented before 2004. However, they will be required to negotiate licensing agreements in order to copy and sell newer drugs, such as the second-line AIDS therapies. It is not yet clear whether Indian firms will pay royalties for the first time on the older drugs used in first-line therapy.

2. We also computed the costs and cost-effectiveness of treatment if second-line therapy were reduced in price by 90 percent.

3. If second-line therapy falls to 10 percent of its current price, the cost per life-year saved falls to US$940 (B 37,600) per life-year saved under the NAPHA scenario, only slightly more than the cost per year of saving fewer life-years with only first-line therapy. The present value of future ART spending drops from US$5.7 billion (B 228 billion) through 2025 to only US$2.5 billion (B 100 billion) a saving over the entire period of US$3.2 billion discounted dollars (B 128 billion).

4. This result is in contrast to the results of simulation modeling in India, where a reduction of condom use from 50 percent to 40 percent was enough to completely offset all the health gains from ART (Over and others 2004, p. 101). The projected impact of adverse behavioral change or "disinhibition" was worse in India because the epidemic is at an earlier stage and because the authors used a longer time horizon.

# CHAPTER 7

# Major Findings and Recommendations

The central finding of this study is that under the primary set of assumptions, the Thai program to treat AIDS patients will save millions of years of healthy life at a cost of US$2,145 (B 85,800) per life-year. This program is less cost-effective than a similar program with first-line therapy only but more cost-effective than some other types of health interventions for adults, such as treatment for end-stage renal disease or some forms of cancer. Another key finding is that Thailand should enhance its program to encourage early recruitment and to finance universal access to the groups of people living with HIV/AIDS, which can improve adherence.

## Major Findings

### Finding 1: NAPHA with First-Line Regimen Only Is the Most Cost-Effective Policy Option of Those Studied

NAPHA with first-line therapy only—at a cost of US$736 (B 29,440) per discounted life-year saved—is the most affordable and cost-effective policy option modeled in this report. If cost-effectiveness were to be adopted as the single decision tool, then NAPHA with first-line only is clearly the superior policy. However, other considerations may weigh heavily on the government's final decision as to what policy to adopt. From the perspective of this study, affordability and equity are also relevant criteria.

An argument for horizontal equity would compare NAPHA with and without second-line therapy to the cost of saving life-years through subsidized treatment of other adult illnesses, such as cancer, heart disease, or end-stage renal disease. This comparison would show that NAPHA with second-line therapy is cost-effective relative to those other interventions. Advocates of vertical equity would argue that the government should ensure that the people at the bottom of the income distribution have access to care that people in the top one-fifth will purchase for themselves (including second-line therapy).

### Finding 2: NAPHA with Second-Line Therapy Is Still Affordable and Yields Larger Benefits in Terms of Life-Years Saved

By 2015, the current NAPHA policy will have added about 220,000 people per year to the living population. Even at the end of the projection horizon, when the Thai AIDS epidemic is predicted to slow, the NAPHA policy will save about 190,000 life-years each year. Hence, 10 percent more life-years would be saved under the current NAPHA policy than under the an equivalent NAPHA without second-line therapy. By keeping people alive longer, NAPHA will be associated with an increase in the number of HIV-infected people in Thailand, as well as with a significant increase in the number of people living with HIV/AIDS who are on treatment. As a result, prevalence rates will no longer be an adequate objective for national HIV strategy (because success in treatment will be tied to an increase in prevalence rate).

The total cost of NAPHA with second-line therapy reaches a ceiling at US$500 million (B 20 billion) per year in 2008. Beginning in 2010, expenditures on second-line therapy account for more than one-half of total ART spending. By the end of the projection, the one-fourth of patients receiving second-line therapy absorb three-fourths of the treatment budget. The projected cost of NAPHA will increase Thailand's AIDS spending from its current level of about US$100 million (B 4 billion) per year to more than five times this amount in 2020. However, even at its peak, total spending on AIDS treatment will require increasing the total health care spending by less than 25 percent. We judge this level of expenditure to be affordable to the Thai government.

### Finding 3: Policy Options to Enhance Adherence and Recruit Patients Earlier Are a Good Public Investment

Timely patient recruitment and enhanced adherence buy additional life-years. If initiated now, the expanded voluntary counseling and testing (VCT), augmented adherence, and "both" policies would benefit more patients each year until the approaches save, respectively, 18,000, 50,000, and 60,000 additional life-years in 2020, on top of the 210,000 life-years saved that were generated by NAPHA alone in that year. Thus, for 2020, the alternative policies offer the possibility of improving NAPHA benefits by almost 30 percent.

These expanded policies, however, involve additional costs. Of the four policies considered, the current NAPHA policy is the most cost-effective. The second-most cost-effective is the augmented treatment policy, which enhances patient adherence. We estimate that systematically adding patient support groups to all treatment sites in Thailand would increase the cost per life-year saved by less than US$40 (B 1,600), thereby making this a good investment. Under the central assumptions of the model, spending the resources on expanded HIV testing in order to recruit patients in a more timely manner would increase the cost per life-year saved by only another US$60 (B 2,400), which also seems like a good buy. Thus, we recommend that Thailand undertake both of the two analyzed policies to strengthen treatment, bringing the estimated cost per life-year saved to US$2,243 (B 89,720).[1]

### Finding 4: Public Financing Will Help Ensure Equitable Access to ART for Poor Patients

Suppose that Thailand had reduced the price of first-line ART by authorizing the production of GPO-vir but had refrained from subsidizing treatment. For households in the top two quintiles in the income distribution, first-line ART could be affordable through user fees. Even for households in the poorest two quintiles, the US$842 (B 33,680) cost of first-line therapy compares with the medical expenses of the sickest households for a single year. The problems for the poorest households are likely to be caused by two unusual features of the cost of treatment.

- First, the treatment must continue for the rest of the patient's life. For households in the lowest 80 percent of the income distribution that are able to pay US$842 for one year, the second and third years will become increasingly onerous.

- Second, poverty-induced laxity in treatment will lead to treatment failure, to development of resistant strains of the virus, to spread of those resistant strains to others, and to the requirement that the patient move to second-line therapy.

Although it is conceivable that the cost of first-line therapy could be partially financed with user fees, second-line therapy is much more expensive, exceeding total household income of 40 percent of the population. Most people on first-line therapy will eventually need second-line therapy, and they will not be able to afford it without public support.

### Finding 5: Public Financing Can Strengthen Positive Spillovers and Limit Negative Spillovers of ART

ART may be used to increase the effectiveness of prevention activities. However, this beneficial effect of ART requires greater integration of treatment and prevention efforts than currently exists in Thailand.

Poor adherence to first-line therapy will speed the development of viral resistance to those drugs and will hasten the day when the patient must move to second-line therapy. Public intervention to support adherence can limit the spread of resistant virus. From a social as well as an individual perspective, adherence support mechanisms such as the augmented public care we model in this report are likely to be cost-effective as well as therapeutically beneficial.

### Finding 6: If the Success of ART Rollout Makes People or the Government Complacent about Prevention, Future Costs Could Rise Substantially

If the availability of ART is accompanied by a sustained government prevention program and if it leads people to reduce risk behaviors such as injecting drugs and having unprotected sex, then the cost-effectiveness of ART is improved by about 9 percent, and future government expenditures on ART will go down by US$926 million (B 37 million), or by 14 percent.

Conversely, if the availability of ART crowds out government expenditure on prevention and leads people to increase their risk behavior back to its levels in the early 1980s, government treatment expenditure will increase more than threefold, increasing the cost per life-year saved from US$2,145 to US$6,243 (from B 85,800 to B 249,720).

*Finding 7: Future Government Expenditures on ART and the Lives It Will Save Are Highly Sensitive to Negotiated Agreements on the Intellectual Property Rights for Pharmaceuticals*

Because the drugs used in second-line therapy are patented, produced, and sold by multinational pharmaceutical corporations, Thailand must either pay the high prices demanded by those monopolies or exercise its rights under World Trade Organization (WTO) treaties to grant a compulsory license for the manufacture of the drug, subject to negotiated royalties.

Because Thailand stands to gain a great deal from bilateral agreements to reduce trade barriers with trading partners such as the United States, the Royal Thai government may be tempted to relinquish its rights to grant compulsory licenses for AIDS drugs in exchange for proffered trade advantages. The report finds that the cost of such concessions would be large. For example, by exercising compulsory licensing to reduce the cost of second-line therapy by 90 percent, the government would reduce its future budgetary obligations by US$3.2 billion discounted (B 127 billion discounted) through 2025 and would cut by more than half the cost per life-year saved of NAPHA, from US$2,145 to US$940 (or B 85,800 to B 37,600) per life-year saved.

The size of royalty payments that the WTO mandates to accompany compulsory licensing is indeterminate and subject to negotiation. Thailand could enhance its bargaining power vis-à-vis the multinational pharmaceutical industry by coordinating its negotiations with other middle- and low-income countries.

## Conclusions and Recommendations

In its current form, Thailand's NAPHA is affordable. Under the model's assumptions, it is also cost-effective relative to the baseline scenario. Furthermore, although the two enhanced policies we suggest (early recruitment through expanded VCT and improved adherence through PHA community support groups) are less cost-effective, they are still a good bargain, particularly if both are enacted.

Much of the cost of ART over the long term is associated with provision of second-line treatment. One way to limit the potential financial burden is for the Thai government to make explicit the scope of its commitment to providing public ART: is it a limited commitment to provide only first-line treatment, or is it a more open commitment to provide whatever level of treatment is required by the patient? Estimates of cost-effectiveness show that a version of NAPHA that includes only first-line drugs is much more cost-effective, at only US$736 or B 29,440 per life-year saved, than the policy with second-line therapy. However, NAPHA with second-line therapy saves a quarter of a million more life-years.

A second way for the government to limit its expenditures on second-line therapy is to grant compulsory licenses for the manufacture of patented second-line pharmaceutical products. Doing so will require high-level political resolve that is based on an accurate understanding of the costs to Thailand, the health benefits, the budgetary savings, and the trade repercussions of such action.

Another option would be for the government to explore other financing mechanisms for ART, including greater use of user fees and health insurance schemes. In view of the government's commitment to provide free and universal access to ART through NAPHA, any such plan would have to be carefully designed to avoid excluding people from treatment or discouraging treatment.[2]

Although affordable, expanding ART represents a long-term financial commitment that must be integrated into the budget processes. Once the Thai government begins to finance a patient's AIDS treatment, that access becomes an entitlement that cannot be sacrificed to budget cycles without incurring large political costs. Continuing to support existing ART patients for the rest of their lives and absorbing new ones while maintaining other health programs will require a 24 percent increase in the total health budget by 2013. Because no cure for HIV infection is in sight, NAPHA is a long-term government commitment.

The biggest challenge for Thai health policy makers will be to resist complacency and instead build a synergistic relationship between treatment and prevention. This approach may require devolution of responsibility for both treatment and prevention to provinces or lower levels of government so that government units that succeed with prevention will benefit from the saved treatment costs.

Success in rolling out treatment will make achieving the national AIDS strategy objective of less than 1 percent prevalence difficult to attain, because people with HIV will live longer. The first objective of the national AIDS strategy should thus be redefined in terms of HIV incidence, and it should be accompanied by measures to strengthen prevention in light of expected (and already documented) changes in the risk behavior of both the vulnerable groups and the broader population.

The cost of US$2,145 (B 85,800) per life-year saved through ART may be much more than Thailand would have to spend to save life-years with other interventions. The study recommends that Thailand accompany its expansion of the ART program with vigorous investigation of other promising opportunities to improve health cost-effectively. Prime candidates among those alternatives would be inexpensive HIV prevention programs, including condom distribution and peer education. Expansion of immunization programs, of traffic safety and trauma management, of nutrition programs, and of water supply are all candidates for cost-effective interventions that would save life-years at probably much less than US$2,000 (B 80,000) per year.

## Notes

1. These policies to strengthen ART are independent of and much less costly than the decision to finance second-line therapy. They would be even more affordable and advisable if public finance paid only for first-line therapy.

2. Inclusion of AIDS treatment within the "30-Baht" national health care plan, a policy currently under discussion in Thailand, must take into account both the large cost of NAPHA and its uneven geographic distribution across the country. Space constraints prevent an analysis of alternative financing mechanisms for ART in Thailand.

# Impact of ART on Survival

Data on the effect of antiretroviral therapy (ART) on survival are not prolific, and those data that exist are not necessarily directly relevant to the current Thai experience with ART. To model the effect of ART on the dynamics of the Thai epidemic, we must infer from the existing studies a detailed quantitative profile of survival and progression, one that captures not only deaths but also treatment failure and dropout behavior. We first describe our assumptions regarding the rate of progression of patients in the absence of ART. We then show the progression patterns that we have inferred for patients on ART under various assumptions regarding their CD4 count on entry and the degree of support they receive for adherence. We also must assume how patients who make the transition to second-line therapy would progress. Finally, we discuss our assumptions regarding the effect of early recruitment on survival.

## Progression without ART

A seminal study by Rangsin and others (2004) presents survival data over seven years on two samples of Thai men, of whom 235 are HIV positive and 255 are HIV negative. The HIV-positive men are followed from the date of HIV infection up to a maximum of seven years. The HIV-negative men are followed for an equal length of time. The mortality rate among the HIV-negative men was 3.1 percent; among the HIV-positive men it was 32.8 percent—ten times higher.

Table A.1 presents the annual survival data from Rangsin and others (2004) and replicates in columns (7) through (9) the survival statistics they calculate.[1] Figure A.1 shows the graph of the column (9) survival statistics against time. The figure, which is referred to in epidemiology as a *Kaplan-Meier survival curve*, shows the percentage of the initial cohort who remain alive at each date in the future. Note that the curve begins with 100 percent of the cohort at time zero and descends to 65 percent of the cohort after seven years. If the time of death or loss to follow-up were known very precisely for each patient, no two patients would be likely to drop out at exactly the same time, so the curve would be smooth. In most real-life studies, the time of death or dropout is only known within an interval. Therefore, several subjects are often lost during a single interval of time. In the figure this lack of precision in the data is represented by the flat spots in the survival curve. The width of each flat spot represents a period of time over which the subjects are observed. The vertical drop from one "step" down to the next represents the number of subjects who died at that point. Subjects who are followed for part of the study period and then drop out contribute to the statistics on survival until they drop out, but they are excluded from the analysis after that point. If their fate is unknown, they cannot be considered to have either survived or died, so they are simply omitted from the denominator as soon as they are lost to follow-up.

In addition to the survival curve, figure A.1 also presents the statistical 95 percent confidence interval for that curve. The interval is a measure of the accuracy with which one can estimate the survival patterns in the 1990s of the population of all HIV-infected Thai men from this sample of 235 men, assuming that the sample was drawn at random. The interval is fairly narrow at the beginning of the period but becomes wider as the sample size decreases over time.

For the purpose of the projection model, we need to project survival far beyond the 7-year time horizon of these data out to more than 20 years after infection. The difficulty of doing this task with precision is suggested by the fact that the confidence interval in figure A.1 widens to more than 10 percentage points by year 7. Furthermore, the data in that figure were collected at a time when Thai men had less access to good treatment for opportunistic infections than has more recently been the case. Therefore, to construct a plausible survival pattern for Thai people without AIDS in the current decade, we

**Table A.1** Survival of 235 Thai HIV-Positive Men

| Years HIV+ (1) | Alive at start of year (2) | Lost to follow-up (3) | Actuarial adjusted at risk (4) | Deaths (5) | Alive at end of year (6) | One-year hazard (%) (7) | Adjusted one-year hazard (%) (8) | Adjusted Kaplan-Meier survival (%) (9) |
|---|---|---|---|---|---|---|---|---|
| 1 | 235 | 1 | 234.5 | 3 | 231 | 1.3 | 1.3 | 98.7 |
| 2 | 231 | 0 | 231 | 4 | 227 | 1.7 | 1.7 | 97.0 |
| 3 | 227 | 0 | 227 | 5 | 222 | 2.2 | 2.2 | 94.9 |
| 4 | 222 | 0 | 222 | 9 | 213 | 4.1 | 4.1 | 91.0 |
| 5 | 213 | 4 | 211 | 20 | 189 | 9.4 | 9.5 | 82.4 |
| 6 | 189 | 19 | 179.5 | 23 | 147 | 12.2 | 12.8 | 71.8 |
| 7 | 147 | 80 | 107 | 11 | 56 | 7.5 | 10.3 | 64.5 |
| Totals | | 104 | | 75 | | | | |

*Source:* Rangsin and others 2004.

*Note:* Columns (1), (5) and (6) reproduce the first and the two last columns of table 2 in Rangsin. Columns (2), (3) and (4) are interpolated in order to be consistent with the published data in Rangsin's table 2. Column (7) is calculated simply as column (5) divided by column (2). Column (8) makes the so-called actuarial adjustment used by life-tables and by Rangsin. Column (9) applies the standard formula for the Kaplan-Meier product limit survival rate to column (8) and succeeds in replicating the Rangsin calculations.

**Figure A.1** Survival Curve for a Cohort of 235 HIV-Positive Thai Men

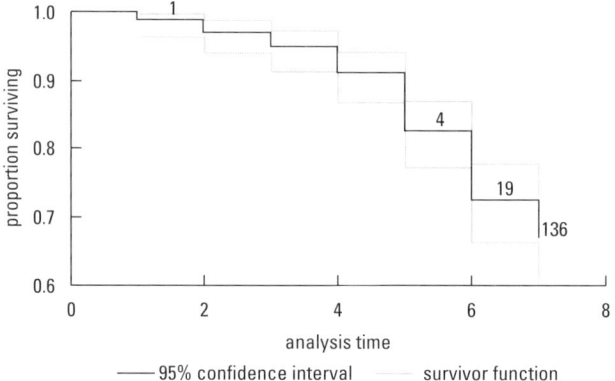

*Source*: Rangsin 2004, table 2.
*Note*: This figure is not identical to Rangsin's survival curve, because it uses the grouped data rather than the original data.

need to adjust a curve based on the Rangsin data to more closely approximate the better survival patterns experienced without ART in other parts of the world. We return to this point in a few paragraphs. However, first we will examine how to use annual survival data like these in a model that projects 20 or more years into the future.

Making a projection of survival beyond the available data amounts to fitting the data to one of several possible functional forms and then projecting on the basis of a choice among these functional representations. The four panels of figure A.2 show the results of such a projection. The panel (a) replicates for easy reference the survival curve from figure A.1. The panel (c) shows the result of fitting one particular functional form, the log-logistic, to the data. Panel (d) projects that log-logistic function into the future with a 95 percent confidence interval. Panel (b) shows how the projected curve and its confidence interval would change if the functional form were the Gompertz instead of the log-logistic.

Note the extreme sensitivity of the results in outer years to the selection of functional form. The log-logistic function is much more optimistic about projected survival than is the Gompertz. At year 10, the log-logistic projects that 41.1 percent of HIV-infected people would still be alive without ART, whereas the Gompertz projects that only 13.4 percent would be alive. We also fit and projected with the Weibull function, which predicts that an intermediate percentage of 33.5 would be alive in year 10.[2]

**Figure A.2** Projecting Survival without ART

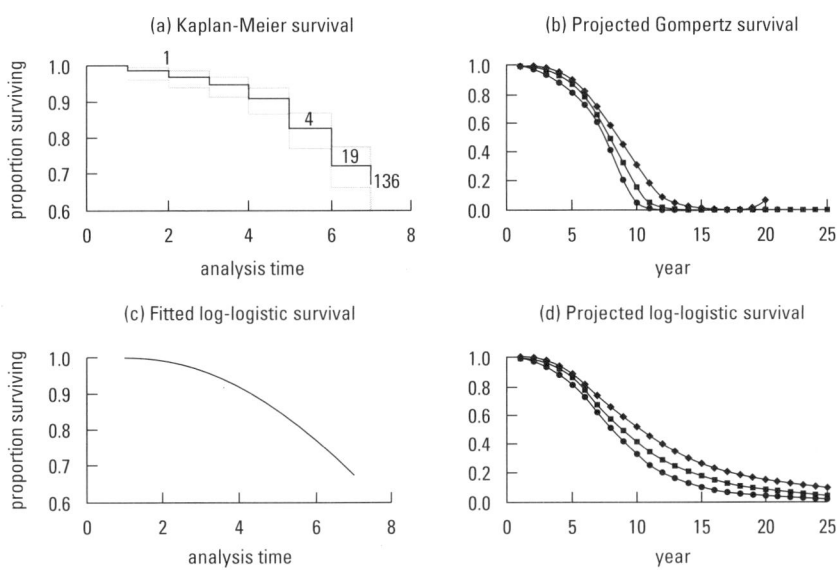

*Source*: Rangsin and others 2004; authors' calculations.

Initial efforts to recalibrate the 1997 version of the Asian Epidemic Model (AEM) to current data used the progression rate without AIDS given by the above log-logistic function fitted to the Thai data from Rangsin (2004). However, projections using this fast progression rate predict that the total number of symptomatic AIDS patients in 2004 would be fewer than 30,000. Because data from the Thai Ministry of Public Health (MOPH) indicate that as many as 40,000 people are currently receiving ART, almost all of whom were symptomatic when recruited, this projection seems to be substantially too low for the current year. From this finding and from the observation that treatment for opportunistic infections has improved in Thailand since the data analyzed by Rangsin were collected, we conclude that the survival experience of patients without ART has recently been better than could have been predicted five years ago from the Thai data.

As an alternative to relying entirely on a projection from the Rangsin data, we turn to the advice of the Joint United Nations Programme on HIV/AIDS (UNAIDS) Reference Group on Estimates, Modeling, and Projections, as presented in their published report (Ghys and others 2004) and in Stover (2002). Figure A.3 compares the log-logistic projection from the Rangsin data with the slow survival pattern without ART

**Figure A.3** Comparison of Survival Curve Estimated from Thai Data with Survival Curve Recommended by UNAIDS Reference Group

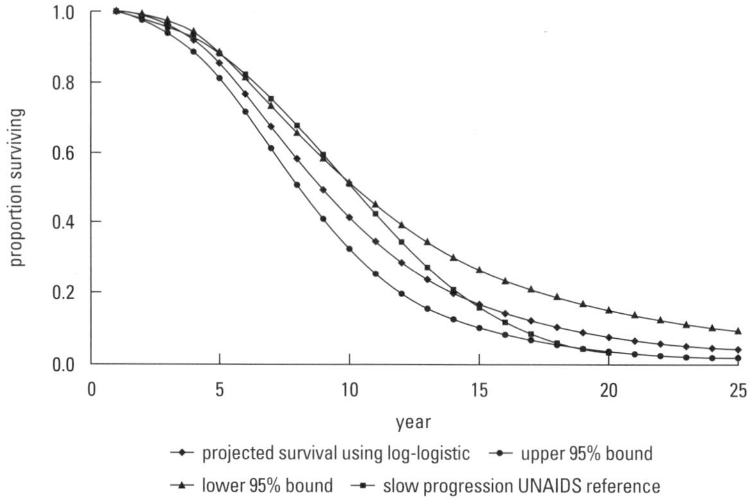

*Source*: Projection and confidence interval are authors' calculations; UNAIDS reference survival rates are the average of the "slow men" and "slow women" rates from Stover's table 2 (2002, 19).

that is suggested by UNAIDS.[3] Note that the pattern suggested by UNAIDS is close to the upper bound of the confidence interval of the first 10 years of the projection from the Thai data and then turns much more pessimistic.

## The Impact of ART with and without Support from Groups of People Living with HIV/AIDS

The existing data on the impact of ART on the rate of disease progression of AIDS patients are summarized in background papers to this report. Because none of the available studies is as complete as the Rangsin data for patients without access to ART, the authors of the clinical background studies have provided, through a partly subjective process, synthetic progression data for each scenario in our simulation model. Table A.2 presents these synthetic data for hypothetical cohorts of 100 patients beginning ART in each of two situations.

Panel (a) of table A.2 presents those lost to follow-up, those moved to second-line therapy (because of treatment failure), and those who

**Table A.2** Synthetic Survival Data on 100 Hypothetical AIDS Patients on First-Line ART in Thailand: Late Recruitment

*(a) Scenario D1 first-line ART without strong PHA groups to facilitate adherence*

| Years HIV+ (1) | Start of period (2) | Length of period (3) | Lost to follow-up (4) | Move to second-line (5) | Deaths (6) | End of period (7) | Hazard per period (%) (8) | Kaplan-Meier survival rate (%) (9) |
|---|---|---|---|---|---|---|---|---|
| 1 | 100 | 1 | 12 | 3 | 10 | 75 | 10.0 | 90.0 |
| 2 | 75 | 1 | 8 | 5 | 5 | 57 | 6.7 | 84.0 |
| 3 | 57 | 1 | 5 | 5 | 3 | 44 | 5.3 | 79.6 |
| 5 | 44 | 2 | 5 | 8 | 3 | 28 | 6.8 | 74.2 |
| 10 | 28 | 5 | 3 | 6 | 3 | 16 | 10.7 | 66.2 |
| 15 | 16 | 5 | 3 | 3 | 3 | 7 | 18.8 | 53.8 |
| 20 | 7 | 5 | 3 | 1 | 3 | 0 | 42.9 | 30.7 |
| Total | | 20 | 39 | 31 | 30 | | | |

*(b) Scenario D3 first-line ART with strong PHA groups to facilitate adherence*

| Years HIV+ (1) | Start of period (2) | Length of period (3) | Lost to follow-up (4) | Move to second-line (5) | Deaths (6) | End of period (7) | Hazard per year (%) (8) | Kaplan-Meier survival rate (%) (9) | Kaplan-Meier improvement (D3–D1) (%) (10) |
|---|---|---|---|---|---|---|---|---|---|
| 1 | 100 | 1 | 10 | 0 | 10 | 80 | 10.0 | 90.0 | 0.0 |
| 2 | 80 | 1 | 5 | 5 | 3 | 67 | 3.8 | 86.6 | 2.6 |
| 3 | 67 | 1 | 5 | 5 | 3 | 54 | 4.5 | 82.7 | 3.2 |
| 5 | 54 | 2 | 5 | 8 | 2 | 39 | 3.7 | 79.7 | 5.5 |
| 10 | 39 | 5 | 2 | 6 | 2 | 29 | 5.1 | 75.6 | 9.4 |
| 15 | 29 | 5 | 2 | 3 | 1 | 23 | 3.4 | 73.0 | 19.2 |
| 20 | 23 | 5 | 1 | 1 | 1 | 20 | 4.3 | 69.8 | 39.1 |
| Total | | 20 | 30 | 28 | 22 | | | | |

*Source:* Gold and others 2005.

have died when adherence is the individual responsibility of the patient and his or her family, without benefit of a supportive non-governmental organization (NGO). Panel (b) shows the improvement in survival and in retention in first-line therapy when a strong NGO, perhaps staffed with volunteers who themselves are HIV infected, helps patients adhere to medication, show up for appointments to have tests taken, and the like. The last column of the bottom panel gives the number of percentage points in improvement of the survival rate attributable to the supportive NGO or group of people living with AIDS (PHAs). The improvement steadily increases from 5 percentage points at 5 years to 19 points at 15 years and then to 39 points at 20 years.

To capture these progression patterns in a simulation model such as the AEM, in which time is measured in tenths of a year, one must interpolate the survival pattern and then compute the survival density for each category of patient. The problem is complicated by the fact that we must estimate from table A.2 the probability of each of the three events that might cause a person to leave first-line therapy. Rather than omitting from the denominator those lost to follow-up, as is the practice in standard survival analysis, we must estimate the probability that a person will leave first-line therapy for that reason, so that we can model that person's return to the pool of HIV-infected people who are not on ART. (The AEM can then return them to the non-ART progression pattern or reexpose them to ART recruitment.) We also need to estimate the probability of a person moving to second-line therapy, so that in scenarios that include this possibility we can model that flow of patients. We must also estimate the probability of death.

Our approach is to treat departure from first-line therapy for any reason as "failure," grouping together the three possible reasons for such a departure. Using this aggregation of the data, we estimate a survival curve without any data censoring. We then decompose the probability of leaving first-line therapy into its three component parts: loss to follow-up, movement to second-line therapy, and death. The results of the initial estimation and its decomposition into the three components is presented in the panels (a) and (c) of figure A.4.

Using the same Delphi-like approach, the authors of our clinical background paper have estimated the progression pattern of 100

**Figure A.4** Progression from First- and Second-Line Therapy with and without PHA Group Support of Adherence Behavior: Late Recruitment

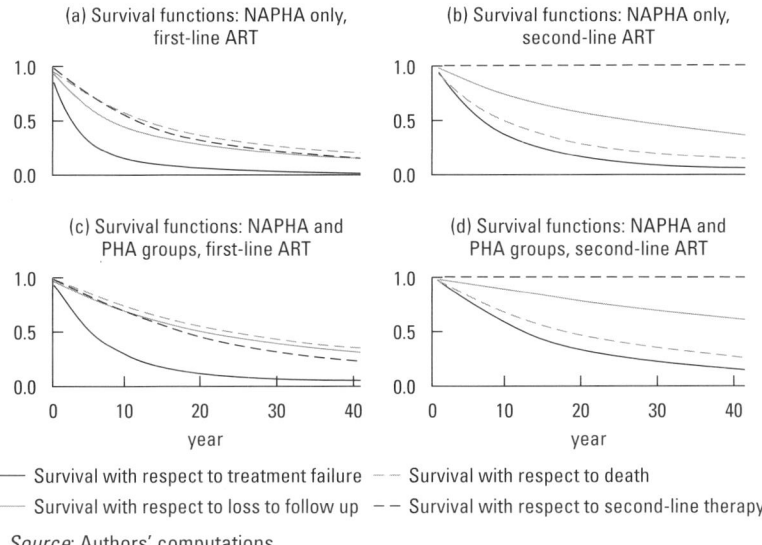

— Survival with respect to treatment failure −− Survival with respect to death
— Survival with respect to loss to follow up −− Survival with respect to second-line therapy

*Source*: Authors' computations.

patients who initiate second-line therapy after first-line therapy failed (table A.3).

## Early versus Late Recruitment

According to the study from Jongkol and others (2004) in Thailand, the median CD4 count for patients entering ART through NAPHA (National Access to Antiretrovirals Program for People Living with AIDS) is 45 cells per cubic millimeter. It is established in the international literature that the success of ART depends critically on the state of the individual's immune system at the time treatment is initiated. See, for example, Hogg and others 2001; Mellors and others (1997). Figure A.5 reproduces the figure from Hogg and others (2001), which shows that the probability of three-year survival drops from 96 percent for those starting treatment at CD4 counts higher than 200 cells per cubic millimeter, to 87 percent for those with counts between 50 and 200 cells per cubic millimeter, down to only 75 percent for those beginning treatment at CD4 counts lower than 50 cells per cubic millimeter.

**Table A.3** Synthetic Survival Data on 100 Hypothetical AIDS Patients on Second-Line ART in Thailand: Late Recruitment

*(a) Scenario D1 second-line ART without strong PHA groups to facilitate adherence*

| Years HIV+ (1) | Start of period (2) | Length of period (3) | Lost to follow-up (4) | Deaths (5) | End of period (6) | Hazard per period (%) (7) | Kaplan-Meier survival rate (%) (8) |
|---|---|---|---|---|---|---|---|
| 1 | 100 | 1 | 4 | 8 | 88 | 8.0 | 92.0 |
| 2 | 88 | 1 | 4 | 8 | 76 | 9.1 | 83.6 |
| 3 | 76 | 1 | 3 | 10 | 63 | 13.2 | 72.6 |
| 5 | 63 | 2 | 5 | 10 | 48 | 15.9 | 61.1 |
| 10 | 48 | 5 | 5 | 11 | 32 | 22.9 | 47.1 |
| 15 | 32 | 5 | 5 | 11 | 16 | 34.4 | 30.9 |
| 20 | 16 | 5 | 5 | 11 | 0 | 68.8 | 9.7 |
| Total | | 20 | 31 | 69 | | | |

*(b) Scenario D3 second-line ART with strong PHA groups to facilitate adherence*

| Years HIV+ (1) | Start of period (2) | Length of period (3) | Lost to follow-up (4) | Deaths (5) | End of period (6) | Hazard per period (%) (7) | Kaplan-Meier survival rate (%) (8) | Kaplan-Meier improvement (D3–D1) (9) |
|---|---|---|---|---|---|---|---|---|
| 1 | 100 | 1 | 1 | 6 | 93 | 6.0 | 94.0 | 2.0 |
| 2 | 93 | 1 | 1 | 6 | 86 | 6.5 | 87.9 | 4.3 |
| 3 | 86 | 1 | 1 | 6 | 79 | 7.0 | 81.8 | 9.2 |
| 5 | 79 | 2 | 3 | 8 | 68 | 10.1 | 73.5 | 12.4 |
| 10 | 68 | 5 | 3 | 8 | 57 | 11.8 | 64.9 | 17.8 |
| 15 | 57 | 5 | 2 | 8 | 47 | 14.0 | 55.8 | 24.9 |
| 20 | 47 | 5 | 2 | 8 | 37 | 17.0 | 46.3 | 36.6 |
| Total | | 20 | 13 | 50 | | | | |

*Source:* Gold and others 2005.

**Figure A.5**  Cumulative Mortality by Baseline CD4 Counts

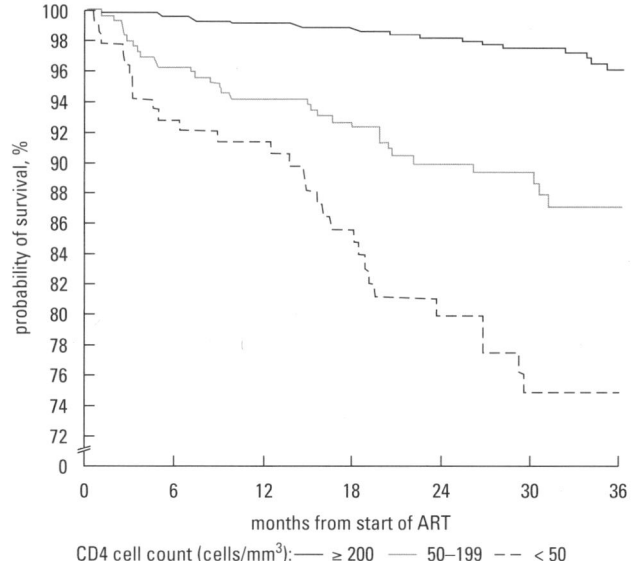

CD4 cell count (cells/mm³):—— ≥ 200  —— 50–199  – – < 50

*Source*: Hogg and others 2001.

## Notes

1.  To replicate the authors' calculations, one must apply the so-called actuarial adjustment.

2.  The median survival times for the three functional forms were ranked in the same way. The most optimistic function, the log-logistic, yields a median survival of 8.89 years, whereas the Gompertz and the Weibull functions yield 7.89 and 8.50 years, respectively.

3.  The slow progression UNAIDS reference pattern in figure A.3 is computed as one minus the average of the male and female cumulative probabilities of death from table 2 of Stover (2002, 19). The greater pessimism of the UNAIDS assumptions in the outer years is probably due to the use of a Weibull function rather than the log-logistic function.

# Costs of Antiretroviral Therapy

Chapter 3 of the text present summary information on the unit cost of antiretroviral therapy (ART), which is then used to construct the projection scenarios that appear in subsequent chapters. This annex gives the background information which was used to construct table 3.9 on the costs of antiretroviral drugs and table 3.10 on the costs of treating opportunistic illnesses, both of which appear in chapter 3. The cost of antiretroviral drugs depends on the exact drugs used, the dosage of each, and the exact price of each drug in Thailand. Since all of these vary across patients, across physicians, and over time, they are subject to continual revision. Chapter 4 analyzes the sensitivity of the book's major results to large changes in the prices of the drugs. Although we did not consider the possibility that the choice of drugs might also change, table B.1 presents the 2004 prices of the individual drugs in Thailand and thus allows the reader to consider the potential effect that specific changes might make to unit costs of treatment.

Successful ART means postponing most of the costs of treating opportunistic illnesses until the time when ART no longer works, a time that comes sooner for some patients than for others. We assume that the patient would fact the same opportunistic illnesses when treatment fails as he or she would have faced had treatment never been initiated. Thus the financial savings achieved by postponing treatment of opportunistic illnesses for a single patient consists of the difference in the present discounted value of treatment between the time ART is initiated and the time ART fails. This savings is larger if the cost of opportunistic illness treatment is larger or if the discount rate is larger. Tables B.2 and B.3 in this annex present data on the distribution of the various opportunistic illnesses within Thailand. Based on these relative frequencies, table 3.10 presents the available data on the cost of treating opportunistic illnesses for the typical Thai patient. These estimates are then used to ensure that projections of the future cost of ART in Thailand properly net out the savings from postponing the treatment of opportunistic illnesses.

One of the most important cost elements in ART is the cost of the CD4 test. A survey of Thai physicians practicing ART, conducted by HIV-NAT for this study, asked the physicians for information on the cost to their patients of CD4 tests. Figure B.1 shows that, despite the fact that NAPHA was more than a year old, there was still substantial variation in the prices paid for these tests. While we have used a moderate value for the cost of a CD4 test in our projections, the Thai government should be aware that some patients are being requested to pay much more or to forego this essential element of good ART.

**Table B.1** Costs of Branded and Generic Antiretroviral Drugs in Thailand, November 2004

| ARV drugs | Strength (mg) and Daily dose | Cost per patient/month | | | | Cost per patient/year | | | |
|---|---|---|---|---|---|---|---|---|---|
| | | Branded drugs | | Generic drugs | | Branded drugs | | Generic drugs | |
| | | Baht | US$ | Baht | US$ | Baht | US$ | Baht | US$ |
| *NRTI* | | | | | | | | | |
| abacavir (ABC) | 300 × 2 | 10,080 | 252.0 | n.a. | n.a. | 35,480 | 887.0 | n.a. | n.a. |
| didanosine (ddI) | 100 × 4 | 1,033 | 25.8 | 50 | 1.3 | 12,400 | 310.0 | 600 | 15.0 |
| lamivudine (3TC) | 150 × 2 | 6,048 | 151.2 | 600 | 15.0 | 72,576 | 1,814.4 | 7,200 | 180.0 |
| stavudine (d4T) | 30 × 2 | 4,146 | 103.7 | 210 | 5.3 | 49,752 | 1,243.8 | 2,520 | 63.0 |
| stavudine (d4T) | 40 × 2 | 4,326 | 108.2 | 270 | 6.8 | 51,912 | 1,297.8 | 3,240 | 81.0 |
| zidovudine (AZT) | 300 × 2 | 4,644 | 116.1 | 1,020 | 25.5 | 55,728 | 1,393.2 | 12,240 | 306.0 |
| AZT + 3TC | (300 + 150) × 2 | 8,340 | 208.5 | 1,500 | 37.5 | 100,080 | 2,502.0 | 18,000 | 450.0 |
| *NNRTI* | | | | | | | | | |
| efavirenz (EFV) | 600 × 1 | 2,319 | 58.0 | n.a. | n.a. | 27,828 | 695.7 | n.a. | n.a. |
| nevirapine (NVP) | 200 × 2 | 1,666 | 41.7 | 900 | 22.5 | 19,992 | 499.8 | 10,800 | 270.0 |
| *NtRTI* | | | | | | | | | |
| tenofovir (TDF) | 300 × 1 | n.a. | n.a. | n.a. | n.a. | n.a. | n.a. | n.a. | n.a. |
| *PI* | | | | | | | | | |
| indinavir (IDV) | 400 × 6 | 4,860 | 121.5 | n.a. | n.a. | 58,320 | 1,458.0 | n.a. | n.a. |
| nelfinavir (NFV) | 250 × 10 | 9,344 | 233.6 | n.a. | n.a. | 112,128 | 2,803.2 | n.a. | n.a. |
| ritonavir (RTV) | 100 × 2 | 2,542 | 63.6 | n.a. | n.a. | 30,504 | 762.6 | n.a. | n.a. |
| saquinavir (SQV) | 100 × 10 | 9,840 | 246.0 | n.a. | n.a. | 118,080 | 2,952.0 | n.a. | n.a. |
| indinavir + ritonavir (IDV/r) | 400 × 4 | 3,240 | 81.0 | n.a. | n.a. | 38,880 | 972.0 | n.a. | n.a. |
| lopinavir + ritonavir (LPV/r) | (133.3 + 33.3) × 6 | 12,692 | 317.3 | n.a. | n.a. | 152,304 | 3,807.6 | n.a. | n.a. |
| saquinavir + ritonavir (SQV/r) | (1000 + 100) × 2 | 11,964 | 299.1 | n.a. | n.a. | 143,568 | 3,589.2 | n.a. | n.a. |

**Table B.1** Continued

| ARV drugs | Strength (mg) and Daily dose | Cost per patient/month | | | | Cost per patient/year | | | |
|---|---|---|---|---|---|---|---|---|---|
| | | Branded drugs | | Generic drugs | | Branded drugs | | Generic drugs | |
| | | Baht | US$ | Baht | US$ | Baht | US$ | Baht | US$ |
| *First line (MOPH guidelines)* | | | | | | | | | |
| 3TC + d4T + NVP | (150 + 30 + 200) × 2 | 11,860 | 296.5 | 1,200 | 30.0 | 142,320 | 3,558.0 | 14,400 | 360.0 |
| 3TC + d4T + NVP | (150 + 40 + 200) × 2 | 12,040 | 301.0 | 1,320 | 33.0 | 144,480 | 3,612.0 | 15,840 | 396.0 |
| d4T + 3TC + EFV | (40 + 150) × 2 + 600 × 1 | 12,513 | 312.8 | 2,579 | 64.5 | 150,156 | 3,753.9 | 30,948 | 773.7 |
| AZT + 3TC + EFV | (300 + 150) × 2 + 600 × 1 | 10,006 | 250.2 | 3,819 | 95.5 | 120,072 | 3,001.8 | 45,828 | 1,145.7 |
| AZT + 3TC + NVP | (300 + 150 + 200) × 2 | 17,684 | 442.1 | 2,400 | 60.0 | 212,208 | 5,305.2 | 28,800 | 720.0 |
| d4T + 3TC + IDV/r | 30/40 + 150 + 800/100 | 13,434 | 335.9 | 3,500 | 87.5 | 161,208 | 4,030.2 | 42,000 | 1,050.0 |
| AZT + 3TC + IDV/r | 300 + 150 + 800/100 | 21,032 | 525.8 | 4,740 | 118.5 | 252,384 | 6,309.6 | 56,880 | 1,422.0 |
| *Second line (HIV-NAT)* | | | | | | | | | |
| IDV + RTV + EFV | 800 + 100 + 600 | 9,721 | 243.0 | | | 116,652 | 2,916.3 | | |
| IDV + RTV + AZT + 3T C | 800 + 100 + 200/300 + 150 | 8,902 | 222.6 | | | 106,824 | 2,670.6 | | |
| *Second line (WHO guideline)* | | | | | | | | | |
| ABC + ddl + LPV/r | (300 + 400* + 1000/100) × 2 | 22,822 | 570.6 | | | 273,864 | 6,846.6 | | |
| ABC + ddl + SQV/r | | 22,094 | 552.4 | | | 265,128 | 6,628.2 | | |
| TDF + ddl + LPV/r | | | | | | | | | |
| TDF + ddl + SQV/r | | | | | | | | | |

*Source:* Bureau of AIDS, Tuberculosis, and Sexually Transmitted Infection, MOPH 2004; Duncombe 2004; GPO 2004; MSF 2004.
*Note:* A daily dose of didanosine in combinations is 400 milligrams once daily for patients who weigh more than 60 kilograms and 250 milligrams once daily for those who weigh 60 kilograms or less.
n.a. = not available.

**Table B.2**  Prevalence of Opportunistic Infections of AIDS Patients at Siriraj Hospital, 2002–04

| Type of infection | Prevalence (%) |
|---|---|
| Tuberculosis | 29.3 |
| Pneumocystis carinii pneumonia | 18.7 |
| Cryptococcal meningitis | 15.7 |
| Cytomegalovirus infection | 6.3 |
| Lymphoma | 6.3 |
| Toxoplasmosis | 5.7 |
| Salmonellosis | 6.0 |
| Cryptosporidium | 5.3 |
| Other | 5.0 |

*Source*: Ratanasuwan 2004.
*Note*: Other includes histoplasmosis, mycobacterium avium complex, PML, candida esophagitis, and rhodococcosis.

**Table B.3**  Opportunistic Infections Presented among 282 WHO Study Participants at 32 Public Hospitals, 2002–04

| Type of infection | % |
|---|---|
| Tuberculosis | 34.7 |
| Pneumocystis carinii pneumonia | 19.0 |
| Cryptococcal meningitis | 15.8 |
| PPE | 13.7 |
| Toxoplasmosis | 3.2 |
| Oral candida | 4.2 |
| Other | 8.4 |
| No data | 3.2 |

*Source*: Supakankunti and others 2004.
*Note*: Other includes penicilosis, chronic fever, and herpes zoster.

**Figure B.1**   Cost of CD4 Counts

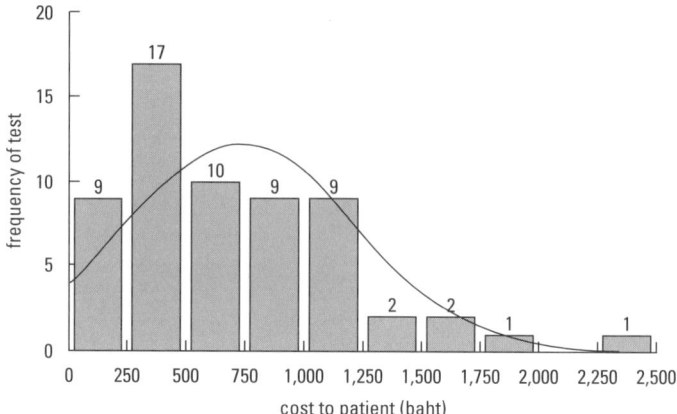

Source: HIV-NAT survey of Thai Physicians 2004.

# Costs of Support Groups of People Living with HIV/AIDS

PHA peer support groups were first set up in Thailand in the early 1990s. In May 2005 800 such groups were active nationwide, most based in public hospitals and supervised by hospital nurses or social workers. In 1998 the Thai Network of People Living with AIDS (TNP+) was formed to coordinate the activities of the different groups of people living with HIV/AIDS (PHAs). The network now has seven offices in different regions of Thailand.

TNP+ began its project to support adherence to antiretroviral therapy (ART) in the Ministry of Public Health (MOPH) ART program in July 2002 (Kumphitak and others 2004). Training and other technical support is provided by Médecins sans Frontières (MSF) and the AIDS Access Foundation: one MSF doctor (10 percent of the time), four full-time nurses, and five full-time social workers. Coordination and ongoing support is provided by 27 coordinators from TNP+ or from nongovernmental organizations (NGOs).

PHA groups are expected to fulfill certain criteria in order to participate in this project. They must have at least two volunteers (the usual number is three) who commit to providing three kinds of service to their clients: one-on-one counseling, home visits, and group meetings. The group must have a working relationship with the hospital staff so that patient care can be planned properly. A budget for PHA volunteer and PHA group activities must be secured. PHA volunteers must be adequately trained in three areas:

- basic knowledge about ART and opportunistic infections
- counseling
- concept of a continuum of care.

In an ideal situation, each PHA volunteer has a caseload of 20 clients, but a volunteer would have fewer if many of the clients are sick and need frequent home visits, if many of the clients are children, or if the area is remote and transportation is difficult. However, because of the rapid expansion of the program and the difficulty of finding enough PHA volunteers and enough budget, many PHA volunteers have a much higher caseload. In May 2005, 150 hospitals had on average three PHA volunteers providing peer support for adherence. In these 150 hospitals, 16,000 PHA are being prescribed ART. Accordingly, the mean caseload of each volunteer is 35 PHA taking ART.

As shown in tables C.1 and C.2, the cost of PHA support per client supported in an ideal situation (that is a caseload of 20 clients per PHA volunteer) is US$78 per year; and in the real situation in May 2005 (35 clients per PHA volunteer) the cost is US$45 per year.

In reality, PHA volunteers carry out other activities, such as home visits for clients who are sick but not yet taking ART. Moreover, the support network of NGO health professionals and TNP+ and NGO coordinators is also actively preparing volunteers from a further 150 PHA groups to take this active role in adherence support for the MOPH ART program. However, the budget for the recurrent costs of the further PHA peer support for adherence has not yet been secured.

**Table C.1** Costs of PHA Support Groups in Thailand: Management Level

*Costs of PHA Peer Support Groups*

*Management Level*

*1) Investment cost of PHA coordinating network (unit: per 300 PHA groups)*

| Currency Exchange Rate | |
|---|---|
| Baht | US$ |
| 40 | 1 |
| Discount Rate | 3% |

| Items | | Investment cost | Life span years | % spent on PHA | Annual investment cost | | Annual discounted cost | |
|---|---|---|---|---|---|---|---|---|
| | | | | | Baht | US$ | Baht | US$ |
| *Capital items* | | | | | | | | |
| Buildings | 7 | — | 10 | 50 | | | | |
| Vehicles | 3 | 600,000 | 10 | 80 | 48,000 | 1,200 | 40,945 | 1,024 |
| Computers | 16 | 360,000 | 5 | 80 | 57,600 | 1,440 | 52,758 | 1,319 |
| Office equipment | | | | | | | | |
| Furniture (tables and chairs) | 24 | 3,000 | 5 | 100 | 600 | 15 | 550 | 14 |
| Telephones | 6 | 3,000 | 5 | 50 | 300 | 8 | 275 | 7 |
| Printers | 12 | 4,000 | 5 | 100 | 800 | 20 | 733 | 18 |
| Photocopy machine | 1 | 40,000 | 5 | 50 | 4,000 | 100 | 3,664 | 92 |
| **Total** | | | | | **111,300** | **2,783** | **98,924** | **2,473** |

*Continued on next page.*

**Table C.1** Continued

*2) Recurrent cost of PHA coordinating network (unit: per 300 PHA groups)*

| Items | | Unit | Operation cost per month | Annual cost | % spent on PHA | Annual Recurrent Cost Baht | Annual Recurrent Cost US$ |
|---|---|---|---|---|---|---|---|
| *Recurrent items* | | | | | | | |
| Office space (rental) | 6 | Cost per month per office space | 4,167 | 300,000 | 50 | 150,000 | 3,750 |
| Vehicles (maintenance) | | Cost per month per car | 1,667 | 20,000 | 80 | 16,000 | 400 |
| Computers (maintenance) | | Cost per month | | | | | |
| Office equipment (maintenance) | | Cost per month | | | | | |
| Utilities (electricity, water) | | Cost per month for 6 offices | 13,400 | 160,800 | 50 | 80,400 | 2,010 |
| Communications (phone, fax, mailing) | | Cost per month for 6 offices | 19,800 | 237,600 | 100 | 237,600 | 5,940 |
| Staff | | Cost per month | | | | | |
| Doctor | 1 | Cost per month | 50,000 | 600,000 | 10 | 60,000 | 1,500 |
| Nurses | 4 | Cost per month | 25,000 | 1,200,000 | 100 | 1,200,000 | 30,000 |
| Coordinators | 27 | Cost per month | 10,000 | 3,240,000 | 100 | 3,240,000 | 81,000 |
| Social workers | 5 | Cost per month | 18,000 | 1,080,000 | 50 | 540,000 | 13,500 |
| Drivers | — | Cost per month | | | | | |
| Volunteers | — | Cost per month | | | | | |

*Note:* Costs included in the estimate are for activities to improve treatment adherence (prevention activities are not included).

**Table C.1** Continued

| Items | Unit | Operation cost per month | Annual cost | % spent on PHA | Annual recurrent cost Baht | Annual recurrent cost US$ |
|---|---|---|---|---|---|---|
| *Recurrent items (continued)* | | | | | | |
| Office supplies | Cost per month for 6 offices | 17,500 | 210,000 | 50% | 105,000 | 2,625 |
| Travel/transportation for M & E | Cost per month per person | 3,333 | 39,996 | 100% | 39,996 | 1,000 |
| Vehicles (gas) | Cost per trip | | | | | |
| Accommodation/hotels | Cost per day per person | | | | | |
| Per diem | Cost per day per person | | | | | |
| Meeting/training cost | Cost for 10 (2 day) workshops per year | 500,000 | 500,000 | 100% | 500,000 | 12,500 |
| **Total** | | | | | **6,168,996** | **154,225** |

**Table C.2** Costs of PHA Support Groups in Thailand: PHA Group Level

*1) Investment cost of PHA support group* (unit: per PHA group)

| Items | Investment cost | Life span | % spent on PHA | Annual investment cost | | Annual discounted cost | |
|---|---|---|---|---|---|---|---|
| | | | | Baht | US$ | Baht | US$ |
| *Capital items* | | | | | | | |
| Buildings (1 room in a hospital) | | | | | | | |
| Vehicles | | | | | | | |
| Computers | | | | | | | |
| TV | | | | | | | |
| VCR | | | | | | | |
| Table, chairs, cabinets | 1 set | 3,000 | 5 | 100 | 600 | 15 | 550 | 14 |
| **Total** | | | | | **600** | **15** | **550** | **14** |

*2) Recurrent cost of PHA support group* (unit: per PHA group)

| Items | Unit | Operation cost | Annual cost | % spent on PHA | Annual cost of saff time | Total recurrent cost | |
|---|---|---|---|---|---|---|---|
| | | | | | | Baht | US$ |
| *Recurrent items* | | | | | | | |
| Office Space (Rental) | Cost per month | 12,000 | | 100 | | 12,000 | 300 |
| Vehicles (Maintenance) | | | | | | | |
| Utilities (Electricity, water) | Cost per month | | | | | | |
| PHA Volunteers (2–3 days/week for counseling services) | 3  Daily allowance | 150 | 58,500 | 100 | | 58,500 | 1,463 |

**Table C.2** Continued

| Items | Unit | | Operation cost | Annual cost | % spent on PHA | Annual Cost of Staff Time | Total recurrent cost Baht | Total recurrent cost US$ |
|---|---|---|---|---|---|---|---|---|
| Travel/transportation for home visit | | | | | | | | |
| Vehicles (gas) | 2 | Cost per day per person | 50 | 15,600 | 100 | | 15,600 | 390 |
| Per diem | 2 | Cost per day per person | 150 | 46,800 | 100 | | 46,800 | 1,170 |
| 2 persons for one home visit = 400 baht/day (3–5 client visits) | | | | | | | | |
| Cost for group meetings | | | | | | | | |
| Food and drinks | 30 | Cost per meeting/person | 25 | 9,000 | 100 | | 9,000 | 225 |
| Transportation | 30 | Cost per meeting/person | 25 | 9,000 | 100 | | 9,000 | 225 |
| *Training Items* | | | | | | | | |
| a) Medical (OI + ARV) | 3 | Cost per PHA trained | 1,733 | | | | | |
| b) Counseling | 3 | Cost per PHA trained | 1,733 | | | | | |
| c) Continuum of care | 3 | Cost per PHA trained | 1,733 | | | | | |
| *Total cost of training* | 3 | Cost per PHA trained /year | 5,200 | 15,600 | 100 | | 15,600 | 390 |
| *Total* | | | | | | | *166,500* | *4,163* |
| *Grand total* | | | | | | | *6,434,970* | *160,874* |
| *Total cost per PHA group* | | | | | | | *187,943* | *4,699* |
| *Total cost per PHA trained* | | | | | | | *62,648* | *1,566* |
| *Total cost per client supported per year (ideal: 20 clients per volunteer)* | | | | | | | *3,132* | *78* |
| *Total cost per client supported per year (May 2005: 35 clients per volunteer)* | | | | | | | *1,790* | *45* |

# References

Akin, J. S., D. K. Guilkey, and E. H. Denton. 1995. "Quality of Services and Demand for Health Care in Nigeria: A Multinomial Probit Estimation." *Social Science and Medicine* 40 (11): 1527–37.

Akin, J. S., D. K. Guilkey, P. L. Hutchinson, and M. T. McIntosh. 1998. "Price Elasticities of Demand for Curative Health Care with Control for Sample Selectivity on Endogenous Illness: An Analysis for Sri Lanka." *Health Economics* 7 (6): 509–31.

Auvert, B., S. Males, A. Puren, D. Taljaard, M. Carael, and B. Williams. 2004. "Can Highly Active Antiretroviral Therapy Reduce the Spread of HIV? A Study in a Township of South Africa." *Journal of Acquired Immune Deficiency Syndromes* 36 (1): 613–21.

Bacellar, H., A. Muñoz, D. R. Hoover, J. P. Phair, D. R. Besley, L. A. Kingsley, and S. H. Vermund. 1994. "Incidence of Clinical AIDS Conditions in a Cohort of Homosexual Men with CD4+ Cell Counts < 100/mm³: Multicenter AIDS Cohort Study." *Journal of Infectious Diseases* 170 (5): 1284–87.

Beegle, E., B. Ozler, and others. 2006. "Young Women, Rich(er) Men, and the Spread of HIV." Working paper.

Beji, M., B. Louzir, H. Tiouiri, M. Khrouf, A. Zribi, and J. Daghfous. 1994. "Tuberculosis Is the Main Pulmonary Complication of AIDS in Tunisia." *Tuberculosis and Lung Diseases* 75 (5): 397–98.

Bell, C., S. Devarajan, and H. Gersbach. 2004. "Thinking about the Long-Run Economic Costs of AIDS." In *The Macroeconomics of HIV/AIDS*, ed. M. Haacker, pp. 311–44. Washington, DC: International Monetary Fund.

Brown, T. 2004. "Modeling HIV Epidemics in Asia: Understanding the Past, Altering the Future." Presentation at the 15th International AIDS Conference, International AIDS Society, Bangkok, July 11–16.

Brown, T., C. Gullaprawit, W. Sittitrai, S. Thanprasertsuk, and A Chamratrithirong. 1994. *Projections for HIV/AIDS in Thailand: 1987–2020.* Bangkok: Working

Group on HIV/AIDS Projection, National Economic and Social Development Board.

Brown, T., and W. Peerapatanapokin. 2004a. "Adding HAART to the Asian Epidemic Model." Paper presented at the workshop "Expanding Access to ART in Thailand: Achieving Treatment Benefits and Promoting Effective Prevention," Bangkok, March 18.

————. 2004b. "The Asia Epidemic Model: A Process Model for Exploring HIV Policy and Programme Alternatives in Asia." *Journal of Sexually Transmitted Infections* 80 (Suppl. 1): i19–24.

Bureau of AIDS, Tuberculosis, and Sexually Transmitted Infection, Ministry of Public Health. 2004. Data provided by the Bureau of AIDS, Tuberculosis, and Sexually Transmitted Infection, Minstry of Public Health.

Carpenter, C. C., D. A. Cooper, M. A. Fischl, J. M. Gatell, B. G. Gazzard, S. M. Hammer, M. S. Hirsch, D. M. Jacobsen, D. A. Katzenstein, J. S. Montaner, D. D. Richman, M. S. Saag, M. Schechter, R. T. Schooley, M. A. Thompson, S. Vella, P. G. Yeni, and P. A. Volberding. 2000. "Antiretroviral Therapy in Adults: Updated Recommendations of the International AIDS Society—USA Panel." *Journal of the American Medical Association* 283 (3): 381–90.

CASCADE (Concerted Action on Seroconversion to AIDS and Death in Europe) Collaboration. 2000. "Survival after Introduction of HAART in People with Known Duration of HIV-1 Infection." *Lancet* 355 (9210):1158–59.

Chacko, S., T. J. John, P. G. Babu, M. Jacob, A. Kaur and D. Mathai. 1995. "Clinical Profile of AIDS in India: A Review of 61 Cases." *Journal of the Association of Physicians of India* 43 (8): 535–38.

Chamratrithirong, A., V. Thongthai, W. Boonchalaksi, P. Guess, C. Kanchanachitra, and A. Varangrat. 1999. "The Success of the 100% Condom Promotion Programme in Thailand: Survey Results of the Evaluation of the 100% Condom Promotion Programme." Institute for Population and Social Research, Mahidol University, Nakhonprathom, Thailand.

Christianson, J. B. 1976. "Evaluating Location for Outpatient Medical Care Facilities." *Land Economics* 52 (3): 299–313.

Cissé, B. 2004. "Recouvrement des Coûts et Utilisation des Services de Santé dans les Pays d'Afrique au Sud du Sahara: Qu'en Est-Il de l'Impact du Paiement des Soins de Santé par les Usagers?" Université de la Mediterranée: Aix Marseille II, Marseille, France. Unpublished thesis.

Colebunders, R., and A. Latif. 1991. "Natural History and Clinical Presentation of HIV-1 Infection in Adults." *AIDS* 5 (Suppl. 1): S103–12.

Community Medicine Department, Chiang Mai University. 2002. "A Rapid Situation Analysis of the Provision of HAART to PHAs by the Ministry's Access to Care Program." Ministry of Public Health and Horizons Program and Population Council.

Dukers, N. H. T. M., J. B. F. de Wit, M. Prins, G.-J. Weverling, and R. A. Coutinho. 2001. "Sexual Risk Behaviour Relates to the Virological and Immunological Improvements During Highly Active Antiretroviral Therapy in HIV-1 Infection." *AIDS* 15 (3): 369–78.

Duncombe, C. 2004. "Clinical Aspects of HIV/AIDS Care in Thailand from a Clinical Research and Community-Based Perspective." A background paper for "The Economics of Effective AIDS Treatment: Evaluating Policy Options for Thailand." World Bank, Washington, DC.

Enger, C., N. Graham, Y. Peng, and others. 1996. "Survival from Early, Intermediate, and Late Stages of HIV Infection." *Journal of the American Medical Association* 275: 1329–34.

Farmer, P., F. Léandre, J. S. Mukherjee, M. Claude, P. Nevil, M. C. Smith-Fawzi, S. P. Koenig, A. Castro, M. C. Becerra, J. Sachs, A. Attaran, and J. Y. Kim. 2001a. "Community-Based Approaches to HIV Treatment in Resource-Poor Settings." *Lancet* 358 (9279): 404–9.

Farmer, P., F. Léandre, J. S. Mukherjee, R. Gupta, L. Tarter, and J. Y. Kim. 2001b. "Community-Based Treatment of Advanced HIV Disease: Introducing DOT-HAART (Directly Observed Therapy with Highly Active Antiretroviral Therapy)." *Bulletin of the World Health Organization* 79 (12) 1145–51.

Farmer, P., F. Léandre, S. P. Koenig, P. Nevil, J. S. Mukherjee, J. Ferrer, B. Walker, C. Orleus, and M. C. Smith-Fawzi. 2003. "Preliminary Outcomes of Directly-Observed Treatment of Advanced HIV Disease with ARVs (DOT-HAART) in Rural Haiti." Paper presented at the 10th Conference on Retroviruses and Opportunistic Infections, Boston, February 10–14.

Galvão, J. 2002. "Access to Antiretroviral Drugs in Brazil." *Lancet* 360 (9348): 1862–65.

Gertler, P., and J. van der Gaag. 1990. "The Willingness to Pay for Medical Care: Evidence from Two Developing Countries." Baltimore, MD: Johns Hopkins University Press.

Ghys, P. D., T. Brown, N. C. Grassly, G. Garnett, K. A. Stanecki, J. Stover, and N. Walker. 2004. "The UNAIDS Estimation and Projection Package: A Software Package to Estimate and Project National HIV Epidemics." *Journal of Sexually Transmitted Infections* 80 (Suppl. 1): i5–9.

Gold, J., C. Duncombe, and others. 2005. Background paper for "The Economics of Effective AIDS Treatment: Evaluating Policy Options for Thailand." World Bank, Washington, DC.

Gold, J., C. Duncombe, and E. Masaki. 2005. "HIV-NAT Survey of Thai Physicians, 2004 and 2005."

GPO (Government Pharmaceutical Organization) 2004. "Price Lists of Drugs." GPO, Bangkok, Thailand.

Guest, P., J. du Guerny, and L.-N. Hsu. 2003. "From Early Warning to Development Sector Responses against HIV/AIDS Epidemics." Bangkok, United Nations Development Programme.

Hira, S. K., H. L. Dupont, D. N. Lanjewar, and Y. N. Dholakia. 1998. "Severe Weight Loss: The Predominant Clinical Presentation of Tuberculosis in Patients with HIV Infection in India." *National Medical Journal of India* 11 (6): 256–58.

Hira, S. K., H. L. Dupont, and T. Sirisanthana. 1998. "Clinical Spectrum of HIV/AIDS in the Asia-Pacific Region." *AIDS* 12 (Suppl. B): S145–54.

Hogg, R. S., B. Yip, K. J. Chan, E. Wood, K. J. Craib, M. V. O'Shaughnessy, and J. S. Montaner. 2001. "Rates of Disease Progression by Baseline CD4 Cell Count and Viral Load after Initiating Triple-Drug Therapy." *Journal of the American Medical Association* 286 (20): 2568–77.

Honda, A., H. Miura, T. Yasuda, P. Varophas, S. Lertchayantee. 2003. "Analyzing the Medical Costs of a Package for HIV/AIDS Care in Phayao in Northern Thailand." *JICA.*

Hoover, D. R., A. J. Saah, H. Bacellar, J. Phair, R. Detels, R. Anderson, and R. A. Kaslow. 1993. "Clinical Manifestations of AIDS in the Era of Pneumocystis Prophylaxis: Multicenter AIDS Cohort Study." *New England Journal of Medicine* 329 (26): 1922–26.

Jongudomsuk, P., J. Thammatuch-Aree, and P. Chittinanda. 2003. "Pro-Poor Health Financing Schemes in Thailand: A Review of Country Experience." Working Paper 31009, World Bank, Washington, DC.

Kleeberger, C. A., J. Buechner, F. Palella, R. Detels, S. Riddler, R. Godfrey, and L. P. Jacobson. 2004. "Changes in Adherence to Highly Active Antiretroviral Therapy Medications in the Multicenter AIDS Cohort Study." *AIDS* 18 (4): 683–88.

Kongsin, S., S. Jiamton, B. Tantisak, and S. Thanprasertsuk. 2004. "Comparison of Public and Private Cost of Opportunistic Infection: Experience from Thailand." Abstract presented at the 15th International AIDS Conference, Bangkok, July 11–16.

Krentz, H. B., M. C. Auld, and M. J. Gill. 2004. "The High Cost of Medical Care for Patients Who Present Late (CD4 <200 cells/microL) with HIV Infection." *HIV Medicine* 5 (2): 93–98.

Kumphitak, A., S. Kasi-Sedapan, D. Wilson, N. Ford, P. Adpoon, S. Kaetkaew, J. Praemchaiporn, A. Sae-Lim, S. Tapa, S. Teemanka, N. Tienudom, and K. Upakaew. 2004. "Involvement of People Living with HIV/AIDS in Treatment Preparedness in Thailand: Case Study." World Health Organization, Geneva.

Kunanusont, C., W. Phoolcharoen, and W. Rojanapitayakorn. 1995. "The Preliminary Report on Formulating Rational Use of Antiretrovirals in Thailand." *Thai AIDS Journal* 7: 190–201.

Lanjewar, D. N., B. S. Anand, R. Genta, M. B. Maheshwari, M. A. Ansari, S. K. Hira, and H. L. DuPont. 1996. "Major Differences in the Spectrum of Gastrointestinal Infections Associated with AIDS in India versus the West: An Autopsy Study." *Journal of Clinical Infectious Diseases* 23 (3): 482–85.

Lertiendumrong, J., C. Yenjitr, and V. Tangcharoensathien. 2004. "Cost and Consequence of ART Policy in Thailand." Background paper for the Economics of Effective AIDS Treatment: Evaluating Policy Options for Thailand. World Bank, Washington, DC.

Leusaree, T., K. Srithanaviboonchai, S. Chanmangkang, L. Ying-Ru, and C. Natpratan. 2002. "The Feasibility of HAART in a Northern Thai Cohort: 2000–2001." Paper presented at the 14th International AIDS Conference, Barcelona, Spain, July 7–12.

Levi, G. C., and M. A. Vitoria. 2002. "Fighting against AIDS: The Brazilian Experience." *AIDS* 16 (18): 2373–83.

Levy, V., and J. M. Germain. 1994. "Quality and Cost in Health Care Choice in Developing Countries." Living Standards Measurement Study (LSMS) Working Paper, World Bank, Washington, DC.

Litvack, J. I., and C. Bodart. 1993. "User Fees Plus Quality Equals Improved Access to Health Care: Results of a Field Experiment in Cameroon." *Social Science and Medicine* 37 (3): 369–83.

Marseille, E. 2003. "The External Effects of HAART." Background paper for *HIV/AIDS Treatment and Prevention in India*, World Bank, Washington DC.

Masaki, E. 2004. "Evaluating Financial Implications of Antiretroviral Treatment (ART) Policy in Thailand." Background paper for Expanding Access to ART in Thailand, World Bank, Washington, DC.

Masaki, E., D. Wilson, and others. 2005. "Costs of Providing ART with PHA Support Groups in Thailand." Bangkok.

McFadden, D. "The Measurement of Urban Travel Demand." *Journal of Public Economics* 3:303–28.

MSF (Medécins sans Frontières). 2004. "Untangling the Web of Price Reductions: A Pricing Guide for the Purchase of ARVs in Developing Countries." MSF, Geneva. Accessible on http://www.doctorswithoutborders.org.

Mellors, J. W., A. Munoz, J. V. Giorgi, J. B. Margolick, C. J. Tassoni, P. Gupta, and others. 1997. "Plasma Viral Load and CD4+ Lymphcytes as Prognostic Markers of HIV-1 Infection." *Annals of Internal Medicine*, 126: 946–54.

MOPH (Ministry of Public Health). 2000. "Evaluation of the HIV/AIDS Clinical Research Network (CRN)." WHO Mission Report, coordinated by MOPH, Bangkok.

———. 2002a. "National Guidelines for the Clinical Management of HIV Infection in Children and Adults." MOPH, Bangkok.

———. 2002b. "Report on HIV/AIDS and STIs in Thailand." Bureau of AIDS, TB and STIs, MOPH, Bangkok.

———. 2004. "Analysis of National Budget and Plan on AIDS Prevention, Treatment, and Control, 1996–2004." Bureau of AIDS, TB and STIs, MOPH, Bangkok.

———. 2005. NAPHA Web site. http://www.aidsthai.org/care.

MOPH and Division of Epidemiology. Various years. "Monthly Epidemiological Surveillance Report." MOPH and Division of Epidemiology, Bangkok.

Muñoz, A., C. A. Sabin, and A. N. Phillips. 1997. "The Incubation Period of AIDS." *AIDS* 11 (Suppl. A): S69–76.

Mwabu, G. M., M. Ainsworth, and A. Nyamete. 1993. "Quality of Medical Care and Choice of Medical Treatment in Kenya: An Empirical Analysis." *Journal of Human Resources* 28 (4): 838–62.

Mwabu, G. M., and W. M. Mwangi. 1986. "Health Care Financing in Kenya: A Simulation of Welfare Effects of User Fees." *Social Science and Medicine* 22 (7): 763–67.

National Statistical Office. 2002. *Thailand Socio-economic Survey, 2002.* Bangkok: National Statistical Office.

Over, M., P. Heywood, J. Gold, I. Gupta, S. Hira, and E. Marseille. 2004. *HIV/AIDS Prevention and Treatment in India: Modeling the Costs and Consequences.* Washington, DC: World Bank.

Phongphit, S. 2004. Behavioral background paper for the Economics of Effective AIDS Treatment: Evaluating Policy Options for Thailand. World Bank, Washington, DC.

Phoolcharoen, W., V. Poshyachinda, C. Kanchanachitra, and T. Waranya. 2004a. "Reversing the Spread of HIV/AIDS in Thailand: Successes and Challenges." Thematic UNDP report, United Nations Development Programme, Bangkok.

Phoolcharoen, W., V. Poshyachinda, C. Kanchanachitra, and T. Waranya. 2004b. "Thailand's Response to HIV/AIDS: Progress and Challenges." United Nations Development Programme, Bangkok.

Phoolcharoen, W., K. Ungchusak, W. Sittitrai, and T. Brown. 1998. "Thailand: Lessons from a Strong National Response to HIV/AIDS." *AIDS* 12 (Suppl. B): S123–35.

Pilcher, C. D., D. C. Shugars, S. A. Fiscus, W. C. Miller, P. Menezes, J. Giner, B. Dean, K. Robertson, C. E. Hart, J. L. Lennox, J. J. Eron Jr., and C. B. Hicks. 2001. "HIV in Body Fluids during Primary HIV Infection: Implications for Pathogenesis, Treatment, and Public Health." *AIDS* 15 (7): 837–45.

Population Council. 2004. "Reducing Drop-outs and Increasing Adherence Rates among PLHA on HAART in Northern Thailand (ART Evaluation)." Population Council, New York.

Prescott, N. 1997. "Setting Priorities for Government Involvement with Antiretrovirals." In *The Implications of Antiretroviral Treatments: Informal Consultation*, ed. E. van Praag, S. Femyak, and A. M. Katz, 57–62. Geneva: World Health Organization.

———. 1998. "Policy Options for Antiretroviral Treatment." In Ainsworth, Fransen, and M. Over, Eds. *Confronting AIDS: Evidence from the Developing World.* Brussels: European Commission. Accessible at http://www.iaen.org.

Punnotok, J., N. Shaffer, T. Naiwatanakul, U. Pumprueg, P. Subhannachart, A. Ittiravivongs, C. Chuchotthaworn, P. Ponglertnapagorn, N. Chantharojwong, N. L. Young, K. Limpakarnjanarat, and T. D. Mastro. 2000. "Human Immunodeficiency Virus-Related Tuberculosis and Primary Drug Resistance in Bangkok, Thailand." *International Journal of Tuberculosis and Lung Disease* 4 (6): 537–43.

Rangsin, R., J. Chiu, C. Khamboonruang, N. Sirisopana, S. Eiumtrakul, A. E. Brown, M. Robb, C. Beyrer, C. Ruangyuttikarn, L. E. Markowitz, and K. E. Nelson. 2004. "The Natural History of HIV-1 Infection in Young Thai Men after Seroconversion." *Journal of Acquired Immune Deficiency Syndromes* 36 (1): 622–29.

Ratanasuwan, W. 2004. "Clinical Aspects of HIV/AIDS Care from a University Hospital Perspective." The Economics of Effective AIDS Treatment: Evaluating Policy Options for Thailand. World Bank, Washington, DC.

Royce, R., A. Seña, W. Cates, and M. S. Cohen. 1997. "Sexual Transmission of HIV." *New England Journal of Medicine* 336 (15): 1072–78.

Selik, R., E. Starcher, and J. W. Curran. 1987. "Opportunistic Diseases Reported in AIDS Patients: Frequencies, Associations, and Trends." *AIDS* 1 (3): 175–82.

Sengupta, D., S. Lal, and Shrinivas. 1994. "Opportunistic Infection in AIDS." *Journal of Indian Medical Association* 92 (1): 24–26.

Sittitrai, W. 1992. "Thai Sexual Behavior and Risk of HIV Infection: A Report of the 1990 Survey of Partner Relations and Risk of HIV Infection in Thailand." Program on AIDS, Thai Red Cross Society, Bangkok.

Stephenson, J. M., J. Imrie, M. M. Davis, C. Mercer, S. Black, A. J. Copas, G. J. Hart, O. R. Davidson, and I. G. Williams. 2003. "Is Use of Antiretroviral Therapy among Homosexual Men Associated with Increased Risk of Transmission of HIV Infection?" *Journal of Sexually Transmitted Infections* 79 (1): 7–10.

Stolte, I. G., N. H. T. M. Dukers, J. B. de Wit, J. S. Fennema, and R. A. Coutinho. 2001. "Increase in Sexually Transmitted Infections among Homosexual Men in Amsterdam in Relation to HAART." *Journal of Sexually Transmitted Infections* 77 (3): 184–86.

Stover, J. 2002. "AIM Version 4: A Computer Program for Making HIV/AIDS Projections and Examining the Social and Economic Impacts of AIDS." The POLICY Project/Futures Gap, Washington, DC.

Suarez, T. P., J. A. Kelly, S. D. Pinkerton, Y. L. Stevenson, M. Hayat, M. D. Smith, and T. Ertl. 2001. "Influence of a Partner's HIV Serostatus, Use of Highly Active Antiretroviral Therapy, and Viral Load on Perceptions of Sexual Risk Behavior in a Community Sample of Men Who Have Sex with Men." *Journal of Acquired Immune Deficiency Syndromes* 28 (5): 471–77.

Supakakunti, S., W. Phetnoi, and K. Tsunekawa. 2004. "An Evaluation of Economic Impacts of Improving Access to Care to Highly Active Therapy (HAART) Program for HIV/AIDS Patients in Thailand." World Health Organization and WHO Collaborating Centre for Health Economics, Chulalongkorn University, Bangkok.

Suraratdecha, C., M. Ainsworth, V. Tangcharoensathien, and D. Whittington. 2005. "The Private Demand for an AIDS Vaccine in Thailand." *Health Policy* 71 (3): 271–87.

Taylor, S., D. J. Back, J. Workman, S. M. Drake, D. J. White, B. Choudhury, P. A. Cane, G. M. Beards, K. Halifax, and D. Pillay. 1999. "Poor Penetration of the Male Genital Tract by HIV-1 Protease Inhibitors." *AIDS* 13 (7): 859–60.

Teokul, W., W. Patcharanarumol, and others. 2005. "Thailand National AIDS Accounts." National Economies and Social Development Board and International Health Policy Program, Ministry of Public Health, Bangkok, Thailand.

Thai Network for People Living with HIV/AIDS (TNP+), AIDS Access Foundation, and MSF in Thailand. 2004.

Thai Working Group on HIV/AIDS Projection. 2001. "Projections for HIV/AIDS in Thailand: 2000–2020." Bangkok: Karnsana Printing Press.

Thanprasertsuk, S. 2004. "HIV/AIDS in Thailand: Current Situation, Successes, and Remaining Challenges." Bureau of AIDS, TB, and STIs, Ministry of Public Health, Bangkok.

Thanprasertsuk, S., C. Lertpiriyasuwat, and others. 2004. "Situational Analysis of the Process for Developing ART Policy by the Royal Thai Government." Background paper for the Economics of Effective AIDS Treatment: Evaluating Policy Options for Thailand. World Bank, Washington, DC.

UNAIDS (Joint United Nations Programme on HIV/AIDS). 1998. "HIV-Related Opportunistic Diseases." Technical update, UNAIDS, Geneva.

———. 2002. "Thailand: Follow Up to the Declaration of Commitment on HIV/AIDS." United Nations General Assembly Special Session on HIV/AIDS, Geneva.

———. 2005. "UNAIDS/WHO AIDS Epidemic Update: December 2005." UNAIDS, Geneva.

Unnikrishnan, S. S., K. Abhayambika, R. Varghese, M. Legori, and Sarojini. 1993. "Clinical Presentation of AIDS—A Kerala Experience." *Journal of the Association of Physicians of India* 41 (1): 38–40.

Van de Ven, P., S. Kippax, S. Knox, G. Prestage, and J. Crawford. 1999. "HIV Treatments Optimism and Sexual Behaviour among Gay Men in Sydney and Melbourne." *AIDS* 13 (16): 2289–94.

Van de Ven, P., L. Mao, A. Fogarty, P. Rawstorne, J. Crawford, G. Prestage, A. Grulich, J. Kaldor, and S. Kippax. 2005. "Undetectable Viral Load Is Associated with Sexual Risk Taking in HIV Serodiscordant Gay Couples in Sydney." *AIDS* 19 (2): 179–84.

Van de Ven, P., P. Rawstorne, T. Nakamura, J. Crawford, and S. Kippax. 2002. "HIV Treatments Optimism Is Associated with Unprotected Anal Intercourse with Regular and with Casual Partners among Australian Gay and Homosexually Active Men." *International Journal of Sexually Transmitted Diseases and AIDS* 13 (3): 181–83.

Van de Van, P., S. Kippax, and others. 1999. "HIV Treatments: Optimism and Sexual Behavior among Gay Men in Sydney and Melbourne. *AIDS* 1316: 2289–94.

van Leth, F., and others. 2004. "Comparison of First-Line Antiretroviral Therapy with Regimens Including Nevirapine, Efavirenz, or Both Drugs, Plus Stavudine and Lamivudine: The 2NN Study." *Lancet* 363(9417): 1253–63.

Vernazza, P., J. Eron, S. Fiscus, and M. S. Cohen. 1999. "Sexual Transmission of HIV: Infectiousness and Prevention." *AIDS* 13 (2): 155–66.

Wannamethee, S. G., S. Sirivichayakul, A. N. Phillips, S. Ubolyam, K. Ruxrungtham, M. Hanvanich, and P. Phanuphak. 1998. "Clinical and Immunological Features of Human Immunodeficiency Virus Infection in Patients from Bangkok, Thailand." *International Journal of Epidemiology* 27: 289–95.

Wawer, M., R. Gray, N. K. Sewankambo, and others. 2005. "Rates of HIV-1 Transmission per Coital Act, by Stage of HIV-1 Infection, in Rakai, Uganda." *Journal of Infectious Diseases* 191 (9): 1403–9.

Weniger, B. G., K. Limpakarnjanarat, K. Ungchusak, S. Thanprasertsuk, K. Choopanya, S. Vanichseni, T. Uneklabh, P. Thongcharoen, and C. Wasi. 1991. "The Epidemiology of HIV Infection and AIDS in Thailand." *AIDS* 5 (Suppl. 2): S71–85.

Wilson, D., and N. Ford. 2004. "Challenging and Cooperating with Government: Community Activities Supporting Access to Care and Treatment for People with HIV/AIDS in Thailand." Background paper for the Economics of Effective AIDS Treatment: Evaluating Policy Options for Thailand. World Bank, Washington, DC.

Wood, E., R. Hogg, B. Yip, P. R. Harrigan, M. V. O'Shaughnessy, and J. S. Montaner. 2004. "The Impact of Adherence on CD4 Cell Count Responses among HIV-Infected Patients." *Journal of Acquired Immune Deficiency Syndromes* 35 (3): 261–68.

World Bank. 1993. *World Development Report: Investing in Health*. New York: Oxford University Press.

———. 1999. *Confronting AIDS: Public Priorities in a Global Epidemic*. New York: Oxford University Press.

———. 2000. *Thailand's Response to AIDS: Building on Success, Confronting the Future*. Bangkok: World Bank.

WHO (World Health Organization). 2004a. "3 by 5 Progress Report, December 2003 through June 2004." Geneva, WHO.

———. 2004b. "Scaling Up Antiretroviral Therapy in Resource-Limited Settings: Treatment Guidelines for a Public Health Approach." Geneva, WHO.

Zhang, H., G. Dornadula, M. Beumont, L. Livornese Jr., B. Van Uitert, K. Henning, and R. J. Pomerantz. 1998. "Human Immunodeficiency Virus Type 1 in the Semen of Men Receiving Highly Active Antiretroviral Therapy." *New England Journal of Medicine* 339 (25): 1803–9.

# Index

**Map 2.1** Prevalence of HIV/AIDS in Thailand by Province

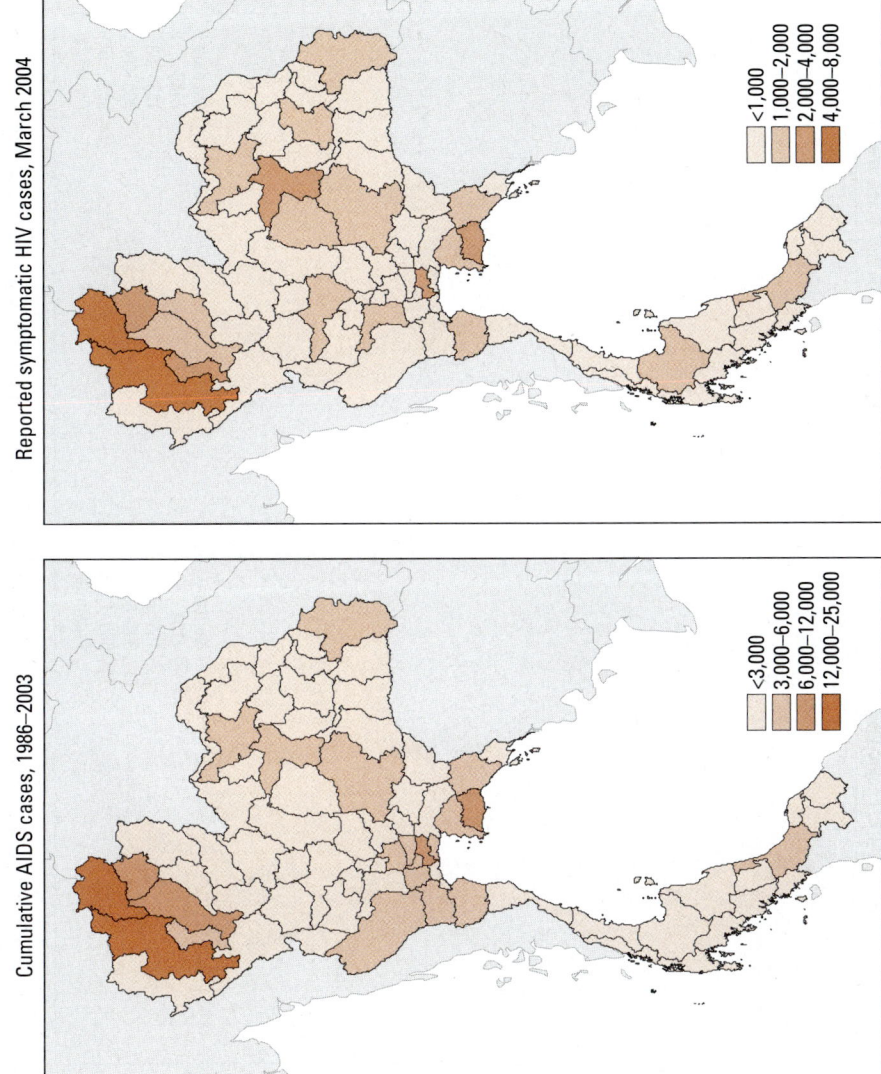

Cumulative AIDS cases, 1986–2003

<3,000
3,000–6,000
6,000–12,000
12,000–25,000

Reported symptomatic HIV cases, March 2004

<1,000
1,000–2,000
2,000–4,000
4,000–8,000

*Source:* Data from Bureau of Epidemiology, MOPH.

**Map 2.2**   Prevalence of HIV/AIDS in Thailand by District

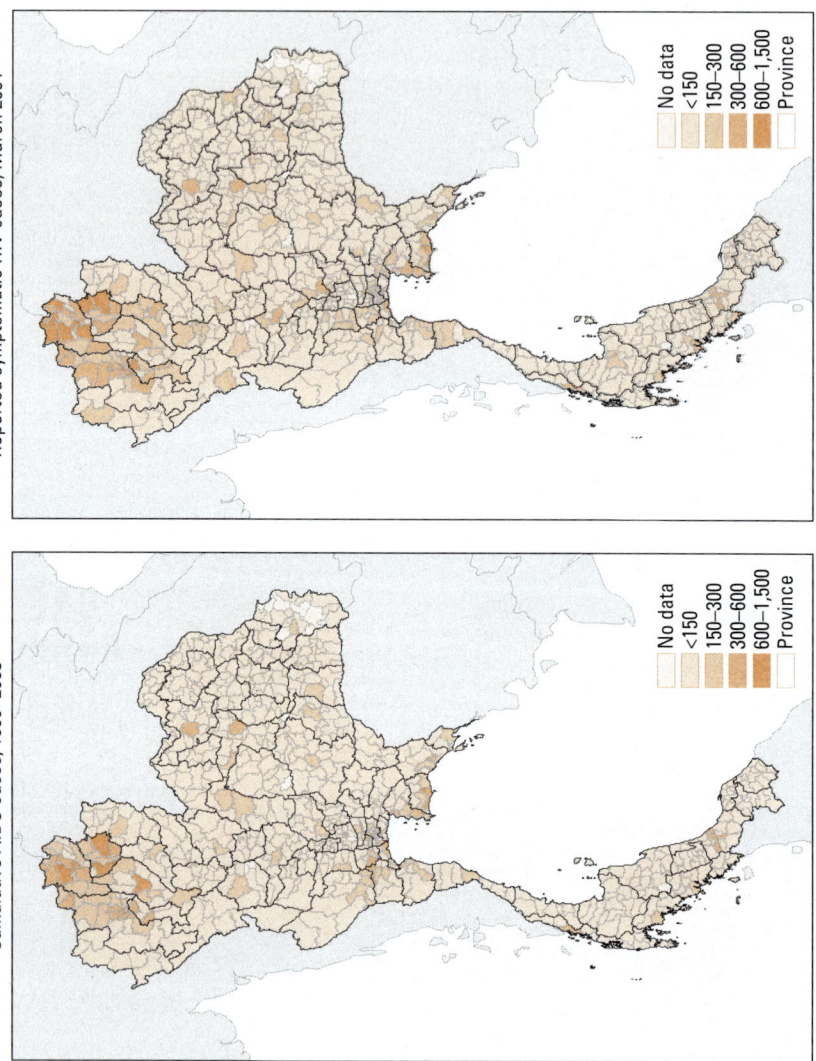

Cumulative AIDS cases, 1986–2003

Reported symptomatic HIV cases, March 2004

No data
<150
150–300
300–600
600–1,500
Province

*Source:* Data from HIV/AIDS and Trafficking Project, United Nations Educational, Scientific, and Cultural Organization, Bangkok; MOPH.

**Map 2.3** Coverage of ART Programs for Symptomatic HIV by Province, March 2004

Number of symptomatic AIDS cases

Percentage of ART coverage

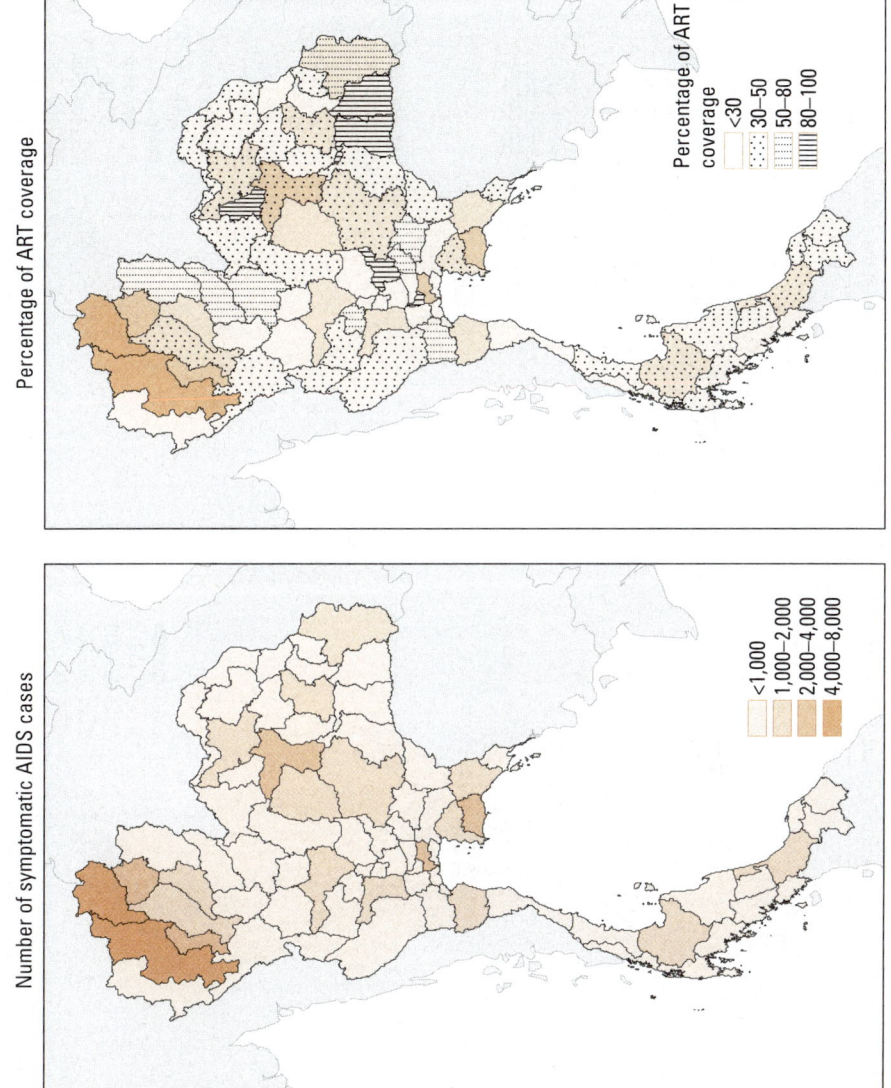

Percentage of ART coverage

<30

30–50

50–80

80–100

<1,000

1,000–2,000

2,000–4,000

4,000–8,000

*Source:* Data from Bureau of Epidemiology, MOPH.

**Map 2.4**  Symptomatic HIV by District- and Province-Level ART Coverage

Reported symptomatic HIV cases, March 2004

ART coverage at the provincial level

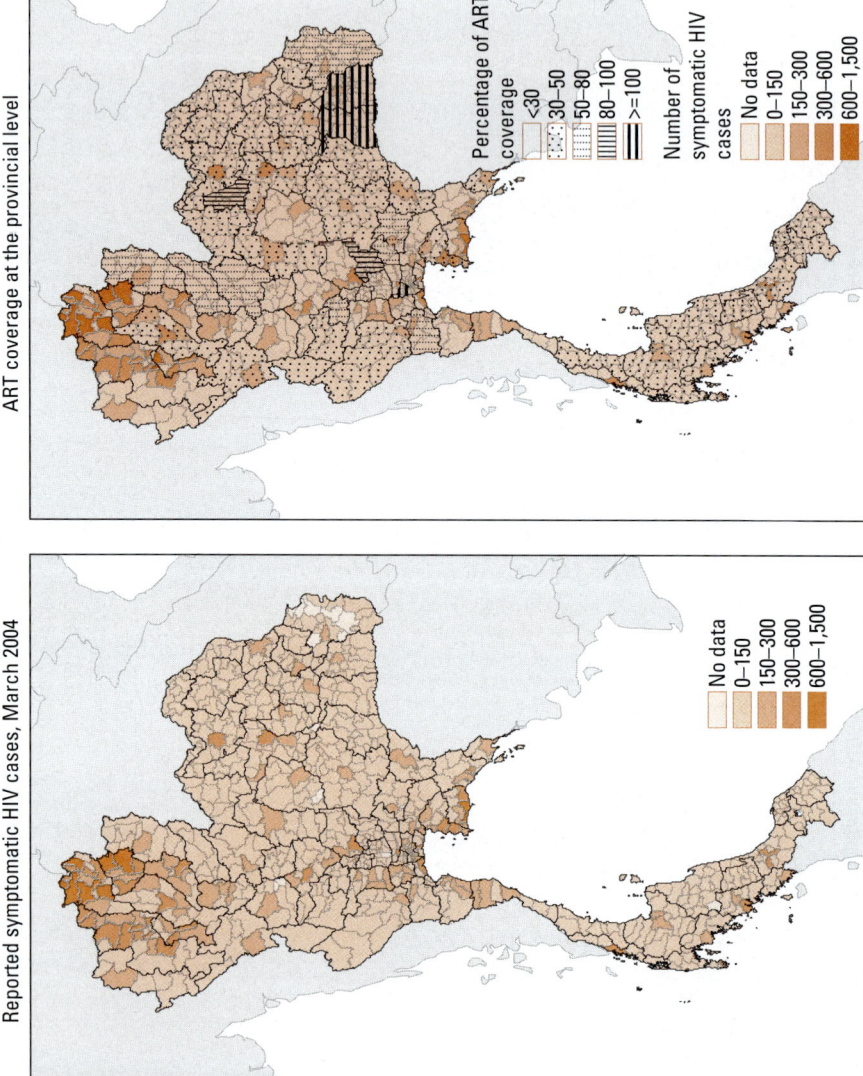

No data
0–150
150–300
300–600
600–1,500

Percentage of ART coverage

<30
30–50
50–80
80–100
>=100

Number of symptomatic HIV cases

No data
0–150
150–300
300–600
600–1,500

*Source:* Data from HIV/AIDS and Trafficking Project, United Nations Educational, Scientific, and Cultural Organization, Bangkok; MOPH. Same as above.

**Map 2.5**   Expansion of NAPHA, 2001–03

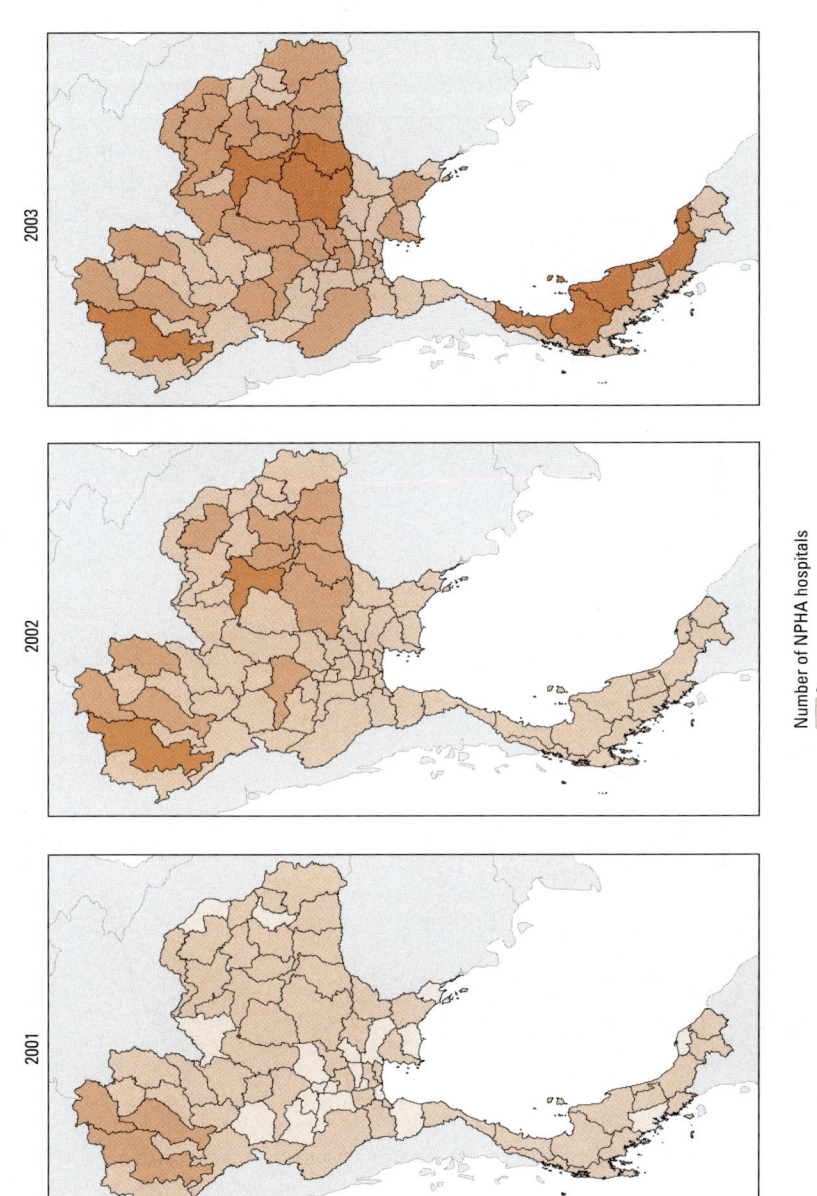

2001

2002

2003

Number of NPHA hospitals

0
1–10
10–20
20–30

*Source:* Data from MOPH.
*Note:* No new hospitals joined NAPHA in 2004.

**Map 2.6    Rate of ART Use at NAPHA Hospitals**

ART participants per hospital

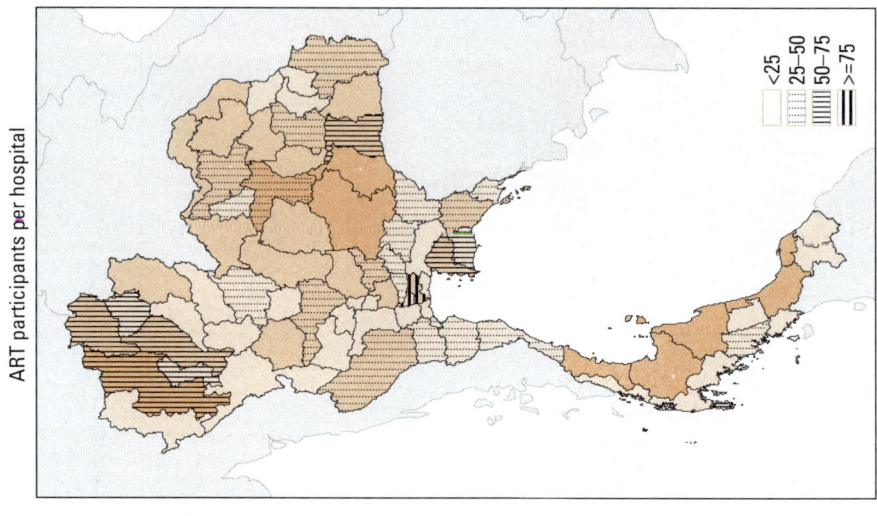

<25
25–50
50–75
>=75

NAPHA hospitals in 2003

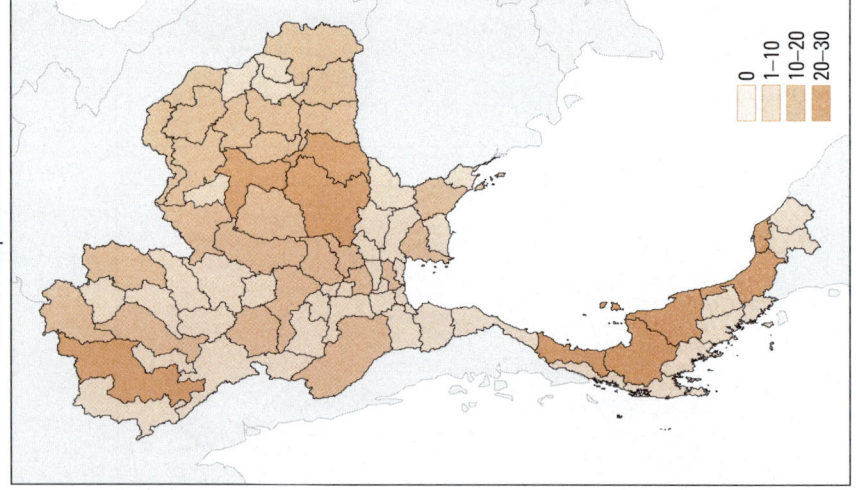

0
1–10
10–20
20–30

*Source:* Data from MOPH.

**Map 2.7**   NAPHA Hospitals and Presence of Patient Support Groups by District, 2004

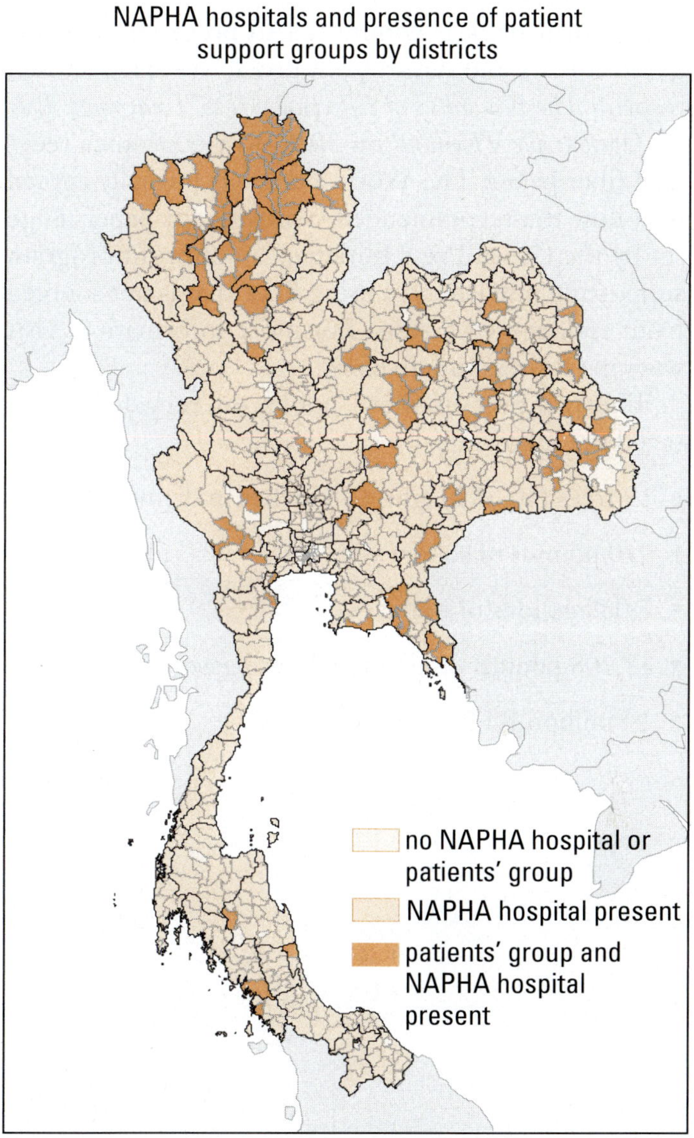

## NAPHA hospitals and presence of patient support groups by districts

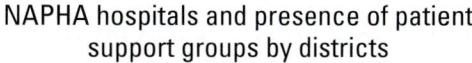

legend:
no NAPHA hospital or patients' group

NAPHA hospital present

patients' group and NAPHA hospital present

*Source:* Data from HIV/AIDS and Trafficking Project, United Nations Educational, Scientific, and Cultural Organization, Bangkok; MOPH.

## ECO-AUDIT
## ENVIRONMENTAL BENEFITS STATEMENT

The World Bank is committed to preserving endangered forests and natural resources. We have chosen to print *The Economics of Effective AIDS Treatment: Policy Options for Thailand* on 30% post-consumer recycled fiber paper. The World Bank has formally agreed to follow the recommended standards for paper usage set by the Green Press Initiative, a nonprofit program supporting publishers in using fiber that is not sourced from endangered forests. For more information, visit www.greenpressinitiative.org.

The printing of these books on recycled paper saved the following:

- 19 trees (40' in height. 6–8 inches in diameter)

- 910 pounds of solid waste

- 7,088 gallons of water

- 11,708 pounds of net greenhouse gases

- 14 million BTUs of total energy

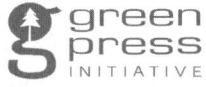